Ophthalmology

OPHTHALMOLOGY
A primer for medical students and practitioners

Calbert I. Phillips

MB ChB, MD, PhD, MSc, DPH, FRCS(Ed and Eng), FRCOphth, DO, FBOA(Hon)
Professor-Emeritus of Ophthalmology, University of Edinburgh; formerly *Honorary Consultant Ophthalmic Surgeon, Royal Infirmary, Edinburgh*

Charles V. Clark

BSc, MB ChB, DSc, MD, ChM, CBiol, FIBiol, FRCS(Ed), FRCOphth, FRACO
Associate Professor of Ophthalmology, University of Queensland, Australia; Consultant Ophthalmic Surgeon, Princess Alexandra Hospital; Director of the Glaucoma Clinical Research Centre, Greenscapes Hospital, Brisbane, Australia

Shigeo Tsukahara

MD, PhD
Professor of Ophthalmology, Yamanashi Medical College, Tamaho, Yamanashi, Japan

With a contribution by

John D.C. Anderson OBE

MA, MB BChir, FRCS(Eng), DO, DCEH (*honoris causa*)
Senior Lecturer, Department of Preventive Ophthalmology, Institute of Ophthalmology, University of London (retired)

Malcolm G. Kerr Muir

MB BS, FRCS(Ed), MRCP, DO, DTM&H
Consultant Ophthalmologist, St Thomas' Hospital, London.

Baillière Tindall
London Philadelphia Toronto Sydney Tokyo

Baillière Tindall
W. B. Saunders

24–28 Oval Road
London NW1 7DX

The Curtis Center
Independence Square West
Philadelphia, PA 19106–3399, USA

Harcourt Brace & Company
55 Horner Avenue
Toronto, Ontario, M8Z 4X6, Canada

Harcourt Brace & Company, Australia
30–52 Smidmore Street
Marrickville
NSW 2204, Australia

Harcourt Brace, Japan
Ichibancho Central Building,
22–1 Ichibancho
Chiyoda-ku, Tokyo 102, Japan

A catalogue record for this book is available from the British Library

ISBN 0–7020–1609–8

Typeset by Action Typesetting Limited, Gloucester
Printed in Hong Kong

CONTENTS

(erosion) ● Chemical burns ● Concussion ● Penetrating injuries ● Sympathetic ophthalmitis ● Enucleation and artificial eyes

PREFACE

This short volume is designed for the undergraduate medical student, general practitioner, casualty officer, general physician, neurologist and neurosurgeon in all countries, but the optometrist, ophthalmic nurse, ophthalmic technician, orthoptist and postgraduate trainee in ophthalmology (at least in the first year or so) will find many parts informative. Understanding is an important basis for learning: explanations are given for the pathophysiology of disease; and reasons are briefly discussed for different courses of action and inaction, which will be useful for family doctors helping their patients to reach an informed decision.

An important way to learn and practise a clinical subject is to record legibly a careful, sympathetic history from as many patients as possible, perform a selective physical examination, anticipated by the history, arrange economically investigations that are minimally invasive, and make a diagnosis based on probabilities obtained from experience, textbooks, etc. A long-term plan is negotiated with the patient and relatives after explanation and discussion of its risks and the possible alternatives. This book has been written and illustrated in order to assist these processes. Practical information will allow the undergraduate to continue to use it in subsequent practice.

Accordingly, although the book is short, we have tried to make it comprehensive and up-to-date for the needs of the intended readers, with a chapter on tropical eye diseases. Ophthalmology is integrated with other subjects: the patient's general health is at least as important as the 'eye health'. For similar reasons, the fellow eye is at least as important as the presenting eye.

We hope the readers will share our fascination with a rapidly advancing specialty.

ACKNOWLEDGEMENTS

We are grateful to the medical artists Mr Ian Lennox, Medical Illustration Unit, University of Edinburgh, and Mr Terry Tarrant of Moorfields Eye Hospital, London, and the medical photographers Mrs Marion Brannan and Mr Stuart Gairns, Medical Illustration Unit, University of Edinburgh for their skill and generous cooperation. Mrs Marion Marshall has been a very efficient typist coping patiently with the many revisions of the text.

Contributions towards the cost of the illustrations have been gratefully received from William Grant & Sons Ltd, Ferranti Defence Systems Ltd and Rhone-Poulenc Rorer Ltd.

The publishers are grateful to Churchill Livingstone for permission to reproduce some of the figures from *Basic Clinical Ophthalmology* by C.I. Phillips.

GLOSSARY OF SOME OPHTHALMOLOGICAL TERMS

Amblyopia	Reduced visual acuity. Always qualify, e.g. strabismic, deprivation, etc.
Ametropia	The state of having a refractive error.
Anisometropia	The two eyes differ in refraction, e.g. one eye myopic, the other hypermetropic.
Aphakia	Absence of the eye lens, e.g. after cataract extraction, or its displacement from the pupil area.
Aqueous flare	The anterior chamber is not optically empty: protein, usually inflammatory, renders a (slit) beam of light visible.
Cycloplegia; cycloplegics	Paralysis of the ciliary muscle (contraction produces accommodation); drugs that produce cycloplegia.
Dioptre (D)	Reciprocal of the focal length of a lens in metres; e.g. if focal length $= +0.5$ m, power is $+(1 \div 0.5)D = 2D$.
Emmetropia	The state of absence of a refractive error.
Enophthalmos	Posterior displacement of the eyeball.
Esophoria	Latent convergent squint.
Esotropia	Manifest convergent squint.
Exophoria	Latent divergent squint.
Exotropia	Manifest divergent squint.
Exophthalmos	Anterior protrusion of the eyeball.
Fovea (centralis)	Central 1.5 mm (diameter) of the macula, 2.5 disc diameters temporal to the disc.

Hyphaema	Blood in the anterior chamber.
Hypopyon	Pus in the anterior chamber.
Kerato-, kerat-	Concerning the cornea, e.g. keratitis, inflammation of the cornea.
KP	Keratic precipitates: aggregates of white cells on the back of the (lower) cornea.
Limbus	Corneo-scleral junction.
Macula	Central 5 mm diameter of retina.
Miosis; miotics	Contraction of the pupil; drugs that make the pupil small.
Mydriasis; mydriatics	Dilatation of the pupil; drugs with that effect.
Pinguecula	Fatty deposit, usually a few millimetres temporal to the limbus.
Proptosis	Anterior protrusion of the eyeball.
Pseudophakia	The state of an eye with an artificial intraocular lens (IOL).
Pterygium	A 'wing' invading the cornea from the limbus at the nasal side (occasionally also the temporal side), apex advancing towards the centre.
Ptosis	Drooping of the upper lid (strictly, blepharoptosis of the upper lid).
Strabismus	Squint.
Uveitis	Inflammation of the uvea, separable into (a) iridocyclitis or iritis and (b) choroiditis.
Zonule	Suspensory ligament of the eye lens.

PRACTICAL CHECKLIST FOR STUDENTS

Section A

You should **do** the following.

1 Take three full histories and write them down.
2 Go through the full eye examination on at least three patients and write down your findings.
3 Take and record distance visual acuity.
4 Take and record reading visual acuity.
5 Use a pinhole.
6 Test visual fields to confrontation.
7 Examine ocular movements.
8 Do the cover/uncover test.
9 Test convergence.
10 Test the pupillary reactions.
11 Examine and draw at least 20 optic discs.
12 Evert half a dozen upper eyelids.

Section B

You should **see** the following.

I. *Clinical cases*
1 Cataracts (several) and cataract extraction with insertion of intraocular lens.
2 Aphakia.
3 Pseudophakia (i.e. intraocular lens or IOL).
4 Diabetic retinopathy (several).
5 (Senile) macular degeneration.
6 Glaucomatous disc cupping (several).
7 Squints (several) and one squint operation.
8 Meibomian cysts (chalazion), and one incision and curettage.

II. *Tests and special methods of examination*
1   Static and kinetic plotting of fields of vision.
2   Applanation tonometry,
3   Gonioscopy.
4   Amsler chart.
5   Colour vision tests.
6   Hess chart or Lees screen.
7   Shallow anterior chamber (eclipse test).
8   Slit-lamp microscopy.
9   Indirect ophthalmoscopy.
10   Retinoscopy.
11   Syringing of tear passages.
12   Shirmer's tear test.
13   Corneal 'staining' with fluorescein and rose bengal eye drops.
14   Intravenous injection of fluorescein with fundus photography, and several fundus photographs.

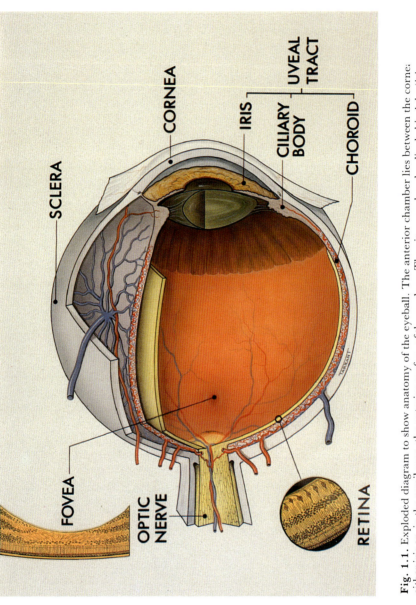

Fig. 1.1. Exploded diagram to show anatomy of the eyeball. The anterior chamber lies between the cornea; either iris or, in the pupil area, the anterior surface of the eye lens. The vitreous chamber lies behind the 'iris-diaphragm'. The fovea is the centre of the macula. See also Figs 1.2, 1.3 and 1.4.

SCLERA

CORNEA

IRIS

CILIARY BODY

CHOROID

UVEAL TRACT

FOVEA

OPTIC NERVE

RETINA

Chapter 1

INTRODUCTORY ANATOMY AND PHYSIOLOGY

Details will follow in special chapters.

The two eyes are like two very small cameras designed to focus rays of visible light on the 'film' — retina — at the back of the eyes, from which images are transmitted to the brain. The cornea and eye lens, especially the former, constitute a powerful lens system. Because the retina lines most of the inner surface of a sphere, a remarkably wide field of vision is achieved.

The two eyeballs are situated in the front of the bony orbits whose margins, especial frontal, provide considerable protection for these two vulnerable parts of the brain. The eyelids contribute to protection by constantly covering a large area of the anterior surface of the globes. Their intermittent closure — blinking — ensures an even tear film on the anterior corneal surface and their reflex tight shutting protects the ocular surface quite efficiently against foreign bodies and other minor injuries.

The normal corneo-scleral envelope, 24 mm in axial length, consists of tough collagen about 0.75 mm thick. To achieve transparency, the *corneal* fibrils are extremely fine and regularly arranged. To allow axons from the retinal ganglion cells to escape from the eyeball and carry messages to the brain, the sclera near the posterior pole is breached at the optic disc. To allow access of rays of light to the retina, the intraocular contents are transparent: the vitreous gel (very fine collagen fibrils in a mucopolysaccharide matrix) occupies about $^7/_8$ of the volume of the eyeball; aqueous humour (very similar to cerebrospinal fluid) fills the anterior chamber and is the only source of nourishment to the lens. The iris, and the lens with its suspensory ligament, separate the anterior chamber from the vitreous chamber. The pupil is constantly dilating or contracting in order to increase (in dull illumination) or decrease (in bright light) the amount of light reaching the retina.

Lining the scleral part of the corneo-scleral envelope is the highly vascular, melanin-impregnated choroid. It nourishes the outer layers of the retina. Anteriorly it continues as the ciliary body, which then continues forwards as the iris. 'Uveal tract' is applied to this series of three tissues — iris, ciliary body and choroid.

The retina, in turn, lines the choroid. Rays of light in the visible spectrum, scattered from objects in the outside world, are brought to a focus on the retina by the lens system of the eye, that is, the cornea and crystalline lens. Some processing of these images occurs in the multilayered retina, from which impulses are then transmitted through the optic nerves to the brain, particularly the occipital (visual) cortex.

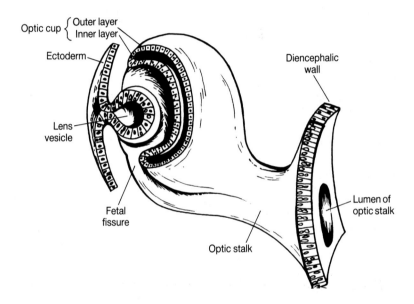

Fig. 1.2. Early development of the eye and optic nerve. It started as an out-pouching from the forebrain, the optic vesicle. Optic stalk becomes optic nerve. Fetal fissure normally closes, but may remain as coloboma of retina; a tiny residue is commonly visible ophthalmoscopically just below optic disc in adults. Outer layer of optic cup becomes retinal pigment epithelium and Bruch's membrane. Inner layer of optic cup becomes remainder of multilayered retina. Lens vesicle is derived from surface ectoderm, hence the association between some rare cataracts and skin diseases.

The retina develops embryologically as an out-pouching from the forebrain, to form the optic vesicle. See Fig. 1.2. That vesicle is invaginated to produce a two-layered optic cup, the outer layer being destined to become the retinal pigment epithelium and Bruch's membrane only, while the inner layer develops into the multilayered retina proper. This results in an astonishing design fault: the light-sensitive layer of the retina is adjacent to the pigment epithelium, i.e. it is beneath all the other layers of the retina! Nature has had to extricate herself from this predicament by making the three layers of cell bodies and three layers of nerve fibres transparent! See Fig. 1.3.

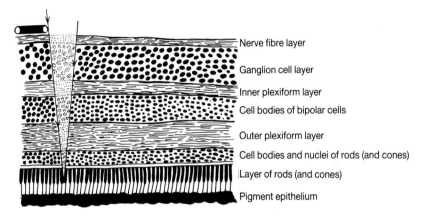

Nerve fibre layer

Ganglion cell layer

Inner plexiform layer

Cell bodies of bipolar cells

Outer plexiform layer

Cell bodies and nuclei of rods (and cones)

Layer of rods (and cones)

Pigment epithelium

Fig. 1.3. Cross-section of retina, the inner (vitreous) surface above. A short length of retinal vessel (top left) is beside the base of a wedge representing rays of light which are brought to a focus at the layer of rods and cones (apex of wedge). Note that the retina has to be transparent because embryonic development has imposed a back-to-front orientation. See also Figs 1.1, 1.2 and 1.4.

Nature designed the macular area, especially the fovea at its centre, to see fine detail by providing it with a high density of, mainly, cones. The peripheral retina has a much lower density of, mainly, rods, so that the brain receives much less detailed information from it. See Fig. 1.4. To minimize scattering of rays of light at the fovea, Nature has shifted peripherally all the superficial layers of the retina, heaping them up just beyond the macula, thereby allowing more freedom of access of rays of light to the cones.

Unfortunately in humans, especially in white races, the inner layers of the retina are not securely attached to the retinal pigment epithelium. The pumping action of the retinal pigment epithelium, which shifts fluid from retina to choroid, is the main factor holding the retina in place. A hole in the retina's inner layers allows fluid to seep into the potential space, which produces a retinal detachment. See Fig. 8.6.

There is a circulation of aqueous humour, quite analogous to that of cerebrospinal fluid. See Figs 5.1 and 5.2. It is secreted by the

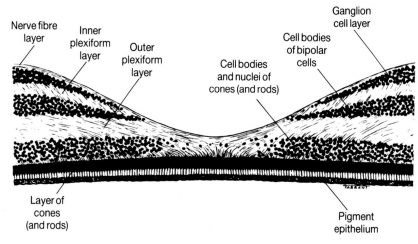

Fig. 1.4. Cross-section of retina at the fovea centralis of the macula, which is the area responsible for detailed vision in the centre of the field. To minimize scattering of light destined to produce a clear image on the cones at the fovea, Nature has displaced other layers of the retina peripherally. See also Figs 1.1, 1.2 and 1.3.

epithelium of the ciliary body, trickles round the lens, between the fibres of its suspensory ligament, then flows through the pupil into the anterior chamber. From the anterior chamber, aqueous humour escapes through the trabecular meshwork into the canal of Schlemm and thence via collector channels into subconjunctival veins. (Arachnoid villi 'filter' cerebrospinal fluid just as the trabecular meshwork 'filters' aqueous humour.) The balance between production and drainage of aqueous humour results in an average intraocular pressure of 16 mmHg above atmospheric. That pressure maintains constant distances between cornea, lens and retina, so important optically. Subnormal pressure is very unusual. Poor drainage of aqueous humour results in a high intraocular pressure (glaucoma), a large subject with its own chapter (Chapter 5).

As for many other organs, there are two eyes. Their movements are coordinated with remarkable neuro-muscular precision. The slightly different images from the two sides, integrated and analysed in the brain, allow great accuracy in the judgement of spatial relations, especially at a close range of a metre or two — stereoscopic or three-dimensional vision. However, a one-eyed patient can manage remarkably well, although he is dependent on uniocular clues for perception of (relative) distances, e.g. size and contour-overlapping, and loses some peripheral field on the blind side.

Chapter 2

CLINICAL ASSESSMENT OF THE 'EYE PATIENT'

Information on methods of assessment appropriate for particular conditions will be found in subsequent chapters (e.g. strabismus in Chapter 4)

Even before taking the history, the experienced clinician, like Sherlock Holmes, will be absorbing details of the patient — age (apparent versus actual), build and bearing, manner(s), dress; before the consultation proceeds far he will ask the occupation (before retirement or before marriage, if appropriate), which may provide an opportunity for a pleasantry to put the patient and escort at their ease. An assessment of the patient's mobility and navigational vision as she enters the consulting room should be included: for example, Parkinson's disease, multiple sclerosis, spasticity, etc. are often more easily diagnosed before the patient sits down. Why is the patient in a wheelchair or walking with a stick? Proptosis, ptosis, facial rosacea, unequal iris colour, etc. may be more easily detected at this stage than when inspection is closer.

History

The importance of history-taking cannot be over-emphasized. The general health is more important than the health of the eye, and the fellow eye is at least as important as the one with presenting symptoms. The history will direct the clinician's attention to certain parts of the eye and adnexa for close attention. As in medicine in general, an experienced doctor soon concludes that a complete detailed systematic history and examination are usually far too time-consuming for most clinical purposes. The same practice applies in ophthalmic history-taking as in the rest of medicine. Make sure your history will be legible and intelligible to others in, say, five years' time. Maximum precision within reason is important. For example, start the history 'The patient had no eye symptoms until . . .' ('Last Thursday' would be obviously silly). When there is doubt, it may be useful to know whether the patient's visual acuity was recorded at school, at work or when obtaining a driving licence. If the symptoms are transient or recurrent, record duration and interval between episodes ('intermittent' means very little). Is the visual defect static or progressive? Which eye or both eyes? Any history of injury? Any family history of eye disease or blindness, especially glaucoma?

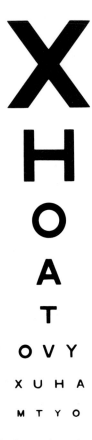

Fig. 2.1. Snellen's test chart. A normal eye can see the top letter from 60 m, the next from 36 m, then 24, 18, 12, 9 (note three letters in that line), 6 m and 5 m. 'VAR 6/18 with spectacles' means that the right eye can only see a line from 6 m that a normal eye can see from 18 m. This particular chart has two advantages: (a) time is saved because single letters are used down to the 6/12 line and (b) all letters are symmetrical about a vertical axis, so that the chart can be used above the patient's head with a mirror at 3 m distance, e.g. in a small room.

Examination

VISUAL ACUITY

Visual acuity is always recorded at the first visit, and most subsequent ones, of a patient with symptoms associated with the eyes, *including especially injury*, and indeed is part of a full general medical examination. Each eye is tested separately, the right always first, to avoid confusing right and left. A Snellen's test chart will already be familiar (Fig. 2.1). The patient is placed 6 m from the chart or 3 m from a mirror in which she sees a chart above or beside her head. She is asked to read from the top. If her visual acuity (VA) is poor and she can read only the top letter, which can be read by a normal eye at a distance of 60 m, then her VAR or VAL is recorded as 6/60 (with spectacles, if worn: always specify); the 6 refers to the patient's distance from the chart and 60 the distance from which a normal eye can read the letter read by the patient. If she reads the top and the next line, her VA is 6/36 ... next 6/24 ... 6/18 ... 6/12 ... 6/9 ... 6/6. Note that 6/6 is of course normal. Many eyes can read one or two lines smaller than the 6 m line; that is recorded as 6/5 or 6/4.

How does one deal with an eye unable to see even the top letter?

- The examiner holds up his hand 1 m or less in front of the patient with two, three or four fingers outstretched and asks 'How many fingers can you see?' 'CF (counting fingers) at 1 m or 0.5 m or 10 cm' may be recorded.
- Worse acuity may allow detection of only 'hand movements' (HM) at 1 m, 0.5 m or 10 cm.
- 'Perception of light' (PL), a positive response to a light shone into the pupil from, say, 10 cm, is the next grade before the final one.
- 'No perception of light' (no PL) is applied to a sightless eye.

Note that in clinics we avoid the word 'blindness', which strictly means no PL although 'complete blindness' would be common usage for 'no PL'.

Do not waste time testing VA without spectacles if a patient has a pair she uses for distance (e.g. TV watching). If she has forgotten to bring her spectacles, or you wish to exclude a refractive error, hold a pinhole close to her eye and she will read down to the 6/12 or 6/9 line unless she has macular degeneration, cataract, etc. See p. 26.

Acuity for reading is sometimes more important than for distance, for example in the elderly with early cataract. The patient must usually wear her reading spectacles, of course, and a good light is important. 'A reading test type' will quantify this accurately (N5 ... N36;

Fig. 2.2), but a newspaper can suffice, at least for an approximation to N8, which is the usual small newspaper print.

For the purposes of the social services in the United Kingdom, 'blindness' means 'so blind as to be unable to perform any work for which eyesight is essential'. In practice, a patient qualifies if her VA is worse than 3/60 in the better eye; if there is severe loss of field of vision, for example due to glaucoma or retinitis pigmentosa, then a better level of VA can still allow blind certification with entitlement to a white stick, visits by a specially trained health visitor, re-training for the young, and a 'blind pension'. 'Partial sightedness' is less precisely defined as 'substantially and permanently handicapped by defective vision caused by congenital defect or illness or injury'.

After recording VA, inspect the lids and eyeballs generally, using the ophthalmoscope as a torch. Include the pupillary light reflex as a routine — if abnormal, check the pupillary near reflex (p. 128). Note any corneal opacities or anterior lens opacities; see Fig. 8.1.

FIELDS OF VISION

Fields of vision need only be tested if a defect is suspected, e.g. because of a CNS lesion, retinal detachment, etc. Although there are many instruments that can be used to plot visual fields accurately (see p. 63), a great deal of information accrues from the following simple test (Fig. 2.3).

- Ask the patient to cover her left eye, holding the upper lid down lightly with the tips of the fingers of her left hand.
- Then ask her to look at the point of your nose or your open *left* eye (shut your right).
- With both your arms outstretched, randomly flutter (noiselessly) your index and middle fingers in the centre of each of the four quadrants of her field, asking her to 'point to the fingers that are moving'. The quadrants are supero-temporal, infero-temporal, supero-nasal and infero-nasal. Avoid the vertical and horizontal lines bisecting the fields: if you test there you will miss a quadrantopia and even an hemianopia.
- Repeat for the patient's left eye. See also p. 63.

Fig. 2.2. Near vision test type, actual size. The patient should, of course, wear (reading) spectacles, if any. Standard print in newspapers and books is usually N8. (Reproduced by kind permission of Birmingham Optical Group plc.)

N.5.

Now we have reached the trees—the beautiful trees! never so beautiful as to-day. Imagine the effect of a straight and regular double avenue of oaks, nearly a mile long, arching over-head, and closing into perspective like the roof and columns of a cathedral, every tree and branch encrusted with the bright and delicate congelation of hoar-frost, white and pure as snow, delicate and defined as carved ivory. How beautiful it is, how uniform, how various, how filling

— numerous renew assurance our sense ewe camera acorn assess cocoa source essence err —

N.6.

how satisfying to the eye and to the mind—above all, how melancholy! There is a thrilling awfulness, an intense feeling of simple power in that naked and colourless beauty which falls on the earth, like the thoughts of life—life pure and glorious and smiling—but still life. Sculpture has always the same effect on my imagination, and painting never. Colour is life.—We are now at the end of this magnificent avenue, and at the top of a steep eminence commanding

— ear race access cannon emu error mace summon season nevermore overawe crane —

N.8.

a wide view over four counties—a landscape of snow. A deep lane leads abruptly down the hill; a mere narrow cart-track, sinking between high banks clothed with fern and furze and low broom, crowned with luxuriant hedge-rows and famous for their summer smell of thyme.

— cam macaroon overseas race ocean excess nurse answer raven —

N.10.

How lovely these banks are now—the tall weeds and gorse fixed and stiffened in the hoar-frost, which fringes round the bright, prickly holly, the pendent foliage of the bramble, and the deep orange leaves of the pollard oaks ! Oh !

— accurse can name one recess oversee own newcomer —

N.12.

this is rime in its loveliest form ! And there is still a berry here and there on the holly, "blushing in its natural coral," through the delicate tracery, still a stray hip or haw for the birds, who

— same accrue car oxen recover ensnare nerve —

N.14.

abound here always. The poor birds, how tame they are, how sadly tame! There is the beautiful and rare crested

— ease on manner even crown cover arose —

N.18.

wren, "that shadow of a bird," as White, of Selbourne, calls it, perched in the middle

— severe room caravan era —

N.24.

of the hedge, nestling, as it were,

— surname seven arrow —

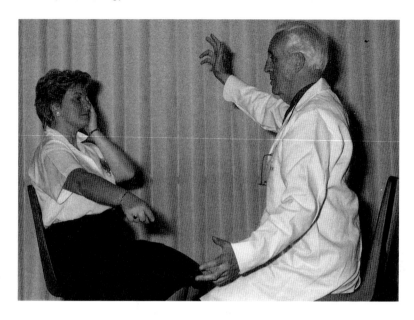

Fig. 2.3. Field testing to finger movements. The patient is asked to 'point to the fingers that are moving'. Note that the test is done in the centre of each quadrant. Only gross defects can be detected such as hemianopia and quadrantanopia.

'Projection of Light'

If her VA is only perception of light (PL), often as a result of cataract, then it is important to check that her retina is intact, i.e. that her fields are full, by testing 'projection of light'.

- Ask the patient to look straight ahead in a darkened room, covering the left eye as above; shine a torch light, preferably with a condensed beam, into her right pupil randomly from the centre of the four quadrants and ask her to 'point to where the light is coming from'. Repeat for the left eye.

Illiterates

Illiterates form a high proportion of the population — e.g. all children under the age of about six years. Pictures of diminishing size can replace the letters on the standard Snellen's test chart. Other methods can also be seen in use by the orthoptists who work in most eye clinics.

OPHTHALMOSCOPY

Ophthalmoscopy is a term applied to seeing the fundus of the eye. 'Direct' ophthalmoscopy would be more accurate here because we will exclude binocular indirect ophthalmoscopy, which is the preserve of the specialist. A few simple tricks will be described to make direct ophthalmoscopy easy, but the most important of these by far is *intensive* practice — as in learning to ride a bicycle or drive a motor car or play golf or tennis.

The ophthalmoscope is a very simple instrument. A beam of light is reflected forwards by a mirror at 45° to the axis of an incident beam of bright light. A peephole in the centre of the mirror allows the observer to look along the middle of the beam of light. Practice is required to find the point on your bony orbital margin on which to rest the instrument so that you can see through the peephole and along the beam.

Dilatation of the pupil by a short-acting mydriatic such as tropicamide 1% eye drops helps greatly; its action is similar to that of atropine, which weakens the sphincter of the pupil (and the ciliary muscle — cycloplegia) by blocking the effect of acetylcholine. Warn the patient that the accommodation will also be weakened for 3–4 hours. (p. 20). The α-adrenergic phenylephrine 2.5% or even 10% will improve mydriasis, e.g. of a brown or elderly iris, by stimulating the dilator muscle of the pupil. *Avoid mydriasis in the rare eye (extremely rare under 50–60 years) with a shallow anterior chamber and small-diameter cornea (p. 66) and a positive eclipse test (p. 71) because of the risk of precipitating acute closed-angle glaucoma (CAG) in it (p. 70).* Before instilling a mydriatic, ask every patient whether a parent or a sibling has ever had an emergency eye operation (excluding one following injury, of course), because that suggests acute closed-angle glaucoma to which your patient may well also have inherited a predisposition (p. 66). Recovery from that mydriasis and paresis of accommodation will take 3–4 hours normally but can be hastened by pilocarpine 0.5% to stimulate the sphincter of the pupil and the ciliary muscle by a direct action on the muscle cells, and thymoxamine 0.5% which is a quick-acting α-adrenergic blocker. Both of these are useful for patients returning to work or who *unavoidably* have to drive a car (*very* carefully) after the consultation. Note that myopes are at negligible risk of acute CAG from mydriatics because they have deep anterior chambers. All these drugs are available in a single-dose formulation that prevents cross-infection. The student should try a mydriatic/cycloplegic for himself in one eye to experience acute transient presbyopia (p. 20).

Use your right eye to examine the patient's right eye, standing on the patient's right side (Fig. 2.4); use your left eye for the patient's left eye,

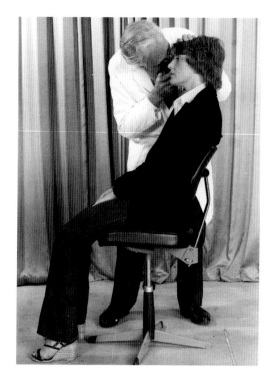

(a)

(b)

Fig. 2.4. (a) The ophthalmoscopist stands *to the side* of the patient, using his right eye to see the patient's right fundus and vice versa. (b) His left hand is placed on top of the patient's head so that his left thumb lifts up the right upper lid, *and* the point of his nose rests on the bent knuckle of that thumb to keep his eye plus ophthalmoscope at the best distance from the patient's eye.

standing on the patient's left side. *Always examine the right eye (ear, leg, etc.) first even if it is the normal one: by that means you will avoid the potential disaster of mixing up right and left; when you go to write down your findings, you will remember what you saw in the first eye and the second eye, not the right and the left (until you are very experienced). Perhaps a left-handed student should examine the left side first?* Watch an experienced ophthalmoscopist at work. If you are one-eyed you will have to use your only good eye, of course: turn the ophthalmoscope upside down, or lean across the patient when necessary, or, with the patient lying on a couch, examine from behind her head (Fig. 2.5).

USE OF THE OPHTHALMOSCOPE

The use of the ophthalmoscope will be described in two rather separate parts in order to emphasize the value of Part I in the diagnosis of early cataract, which is often forgotten (see Fig. 8.2).

Part I

- Put a 0 (zero) lens in the peephole, or your own distance-correcting lens if you are ametropic.
- Apply the ophthalmoscope to your eye and look through the peephole.
- From a distance of half-an-arm's-length (about 0.33 or 0.5 m), direct the ophthalmoscope's beam into the patient's pupil. A dense black silhouette on the background of the usual red reflex will diagnose early cataract (or very occasionally a slight corneal opacity).
- If in doubt, approach to, say, 10 cm from the patient's eye.

Do not be misled by greyish shadows, especially if the pupil is dilated, which are discontinuities in the refractive index of the peripheral lens. Also, you may be confused by an image of the retinal blood vessels, which at this stage you should ignore: move your head-plus-ophthalmoscope quite large distances to keep these images moving so that you can concentrate on any *static* black silhouettes (see Fig. 8.2).

This examination may also reveal vitreous opacities (usually 'floaters') and even slight corneal opacities. The presence of the latter is easily confirmed by focal illumination, i.e. the observer shines a bright light on the eye and comes close for a careful inspection. *Parallax* will also help to decide the site of an opacity (see Fig. 2.6). If the ophthalmoscope plus observer's eye moves up and down or right and left or obliquely, an opacity at the anterior surface of the lens, i.e. in

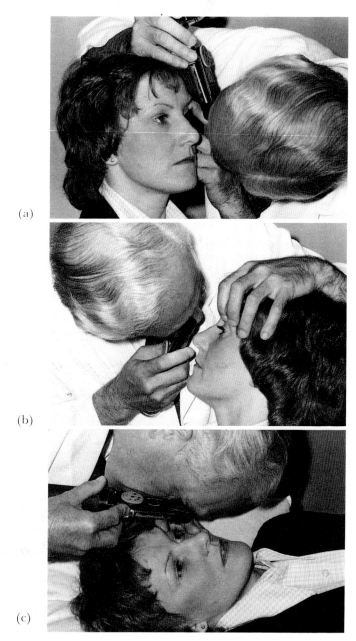

(a)

(b)

(c)

Fig. 2.5. An ophthalmoscopist whose left eye has poor vision can use his right eye to see the patient's left fundus by (a) turning the handle of the ophthalmoscope upwards or (b) leaning across the patient (possibly embarrassing) or (c), with the patient lying on a couch, examining from behind the patient's head.

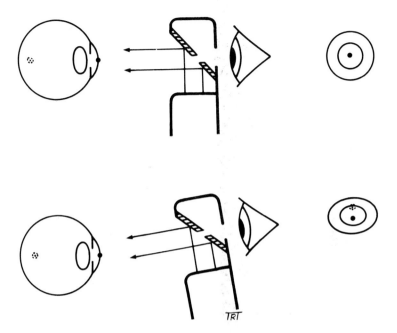

Fig. 2.6. Parallactic displacement reveals the position of an opacity in the transparent media of the eye. The observer's eye should be about 0.5 m from the patient's eye. The upper series of three diagrams shows that an opacity in the visual axis at any depth (left-hand diagram) will appear to the ophthalmoscopist (middle diagram) to be in the centre of the pupil (right-hand diagram). In the lower series, the observer has moved about 10 cm upwards so that he can look *downwards* into the eye: a central corneal opacity (solid dot) will appear to move *downwards* in relation to the pupil, whereas the vitreous opacity (stippled dot) will appear to move upwards; a central opacity at the back of the eye lens (not shown) would also appear to move upwards, but more slowly than the vitreous opacity. Of course, an opacity in the plane of the pupil, e.g. a small opacity at or just under the anterior lens capsule, will not appear to move.

the plane of the pupil, will not move in relation to the pupil. As the observer's eye + ophthalmoscope shifts upwards to attain a downward-directed viewpoint, a corneal opacity will appear to move downwards in relation to the pupil, whereas a vitreous opacity, or an opacity posteriorly in the lens, will appear to move upwards.

Part II
Part II allows the observer (a) to confirm his part I findings and (b) to see the fundus of the eye. Start with the patient's right eye, using your

right eye, for which the following description will be appropriate. See Fig. 2.4a and b, also Fig. 2.5a, b and c. The tricks to use are:

- *Patient* sits reasonably erect, looking straight ahead at a prominent object at eye level, e.g. a door handle. There should be at least 1 m of space on each side of the patient: the ophthalmoscopist and patient must be comfortable.
- *Ophthalmoscopist.*
  (a) Put a + 12D lens in the peephole of the ophthalmoscope.
  (b) Stance: stand at the *side* of the patient so that a line joining your toes is parallel to the patient's visual axis. Feet should be comfortably apart about 30 cm.
  (c) Position: your left heel should be at the level of the patient's right eyeball. Place your *left* hand on the patient's head so that your thumb can lift up her *right* upper lid, crooking the knuckle of your thumb as you do so. Having placed the ophthalmoscope in front of your right eye so that it looks through the peephole, approximate your head-plus-ophthalmoscope towards the patient's eye so that your nose rests on your knuckle: that nose-on-knuckle trick keeps you at the correct distance. Little movement is possible between the ophthalmoscope and the examiner's head: think of the ophthalmoscope as welded to your head.
  (d) With practice, the above manoeuvres take only a few seconds.

The + 12D lens in the peephole of the ophthalmoscope produces a red blur, unless there is a dense corneal opacity or cataract or vitreous haemorrhage. A partial cataract will produce a black silhouette contrasting with a partial red reflex that may become more obvious when the observer turns the milled knob to reduce the power to a + 10D lens — confirming the result of Part I. He goes on turning the milled knob but concentrates on the view through the peephole (and *not* looking at the lens register, which will be changing to + 9, + 8, + 7, etc.), thinking of posterior lens, anterior then middle vitreous. The racking down process goes on until the observer can just see a blood vessel in the fundus clearly, *at which point he stops turning the milled knob*. (If it is continued, the observer merely accommodates to overcome the negative lenses that follow.) If the examiner and patient are emmetropic, i.e. have no refractive error, a 0 (zero) lens should be in the peephole at this point. Note that the technique of starting with a + 12D lens then progressively diminishing the power of the lens in the peephole ensures that the ophthalmoscopist relaxes his own accommodation.

It is usually preferable for the examiner and patient not to wear spectacles for ophthalmoscopy. If the patient or examiner is myopic, a

– lens (negative or minus) is in the peephole when a clear view of the fundus is obtained. A *highly* myopic patient should wear his spectacles during ophthalmoscopy, which allows the examiner a better view of his fundus. If either is hypermetropic, a + lens (plus or convex) will be in the peephole. The patient's and examiner's refractive errors are additive, including sign: for example a + 3D hypermetropic patient and a − 3D examiner will result in a 0 lens in the peephole, as if both were emmetropic.

Systematic Fundus Examination
A clear view of a retinal blood vessel will have been obtained by now, usually one infero-nasal to the disc. Follow it back to the optic disc, from which all retinal blood vessels radiate.

- *Optic disc,* Assess the disc under three Cs:
    Colour : pink or white?
    Contour : edges clear-cut or blurred?
    Cupping : how big is the cup in relation to the disc?
- *Vessels and related retina.* Moving your head-plus-ophthalmoscope as practically one unit, follow the supero-temporal vessels up and out, the infero-temporals down and out, then the supero-nasals up and in, and infero-nasals down and in. The veins are darker red or blue in colour compared with the red arterioles and have a larger diameter (ratio 3:2). Look for calibre variations, haemorrhages and exudates. However, the best way to diagnose hypertensive retinopathy (p. 99) — rare except for accelerated hypertension — is to take the blood pressure! The best way to diagnose diabetic retinopathy (Chapter 10) is to test the urine for sugar 2 – 3 hours after the biggest meal in the day. Assess arteriosclerosis by feeling the radial and dorsalis pedis arteries!!
- *Peripheral retina.* Scan the periphal retina quickly, unless you suspect retinal detachment (p. 115 and Figs 8.6 and 8.8) or retinitis pigmentosa (p. 199 and Fig. 16.1), etc. Ask the patient to look up, down, right and left while you place your occiput in the opposite direction.
- *Macular area.* Finally, look at the macular area (Figs 1.1 and 8.5), which will be very difficult to see through an undilated pupil because it will immediately contract reflexly. The centre of the macula (fovea centralis) is 2.5 disc diameters temporal to the disc but may be more easily found by asking the patient to 'look into the middle of my light'. It is an inconspicuous, rather granular area of the retina, free from blood vessels: there is a bright spot of light at its centre because the normal retina is concave there and so acts as a concave mirror.

Chapter 3

Refractive Errors, Spectacles, Contact Lenses And Refractive Surgery

---

Introduction to Basic Optics Relevant to Ophthalmology

Refraction is defined as the alteration in the direction of a wave form when passing from one medium to another of a different density. One of the most important functions of the eye is to 'refract' rays of light and bring them to a focus on the retina (Fig. 3.1). In ophthalmology, a 'refractive error' describes the situation where the light rays are not focused on the retina, for reasons which will be explained in the first part of this chapter.

A convex or 'plus' (+) lens will converge rays of light, as shown in Figs 3.2b and 3.4. A concave or 'minus' (−) lens will diverge rays of light as shown in Fig. 3.5. A dioptre is the reciprocal of the focal length in metres. For example, if a + lens brings parallel rays of light to a focus (real image) at 1 m beyond the lens, its power is $+(1 \div 1)$D, i.e. + 1D; if at 0.5 m, its power is $+(1 \div 0.5)$D, i.e. 2D. If a − lens diverges parallel rays so that they appear to come from (a virtual image) 1 m in front of the lens, the power is $-(1 \div 1)$D, i.e. − 1D; if from 0.25 m, the power is $-(1 \div 0.25)$D, i.e. − 4D.

The Normal Eye: Emmetropia (Absence of Refractive Error)

In an emmetropic eye, the axial length (easily measured by ultrasound) is usually 24 mm, but it ranges from 21 to 26 mm. That implies that Nature can compensate for a relatively short axial length by increasing corneal and lens curvatures, and for a long axial length by decreasing corneal and lens curvatures; see Fig. 3.1. The optical system of the eye has to be very powerful to bring parallel rays of light to a focus in so short a distance. The cornea contributes around 45 dioptres compared with the eye lens's 15 dioptres. The anterior corneal surface has the

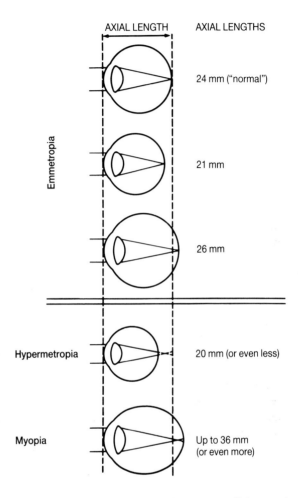

Fig. 3.1. In emmetropia, by definition, parallel rays of light are brought to a focus on the retina, accommodation being entirely relaxed. Note that axial length can range from about 21 to 26 mm so that the eye's lens system 'compensates' by being more powerful in the former and less powerful in the latter, when compared with the 24 mm ('normal') case.

The compensation tends to break down in a short eye to produce hypermetropia (US hyperopia) or long sight, and in a long eye to produce myopia or short sight. Note that, in each case, some compensation has taken place, i.e. the focal point is not at 24 mm distance.

advantage of the big difference between the refractive indices of air and cornea; the refractive index of the cornea and the eye lens differs much less from the refractive index of the aqueous humour and vitreous.

At around 20 mm axial length or less, compensation tends to break down, resulting in hypermetropia; see Fig. 3.1. At more than 26 mm, myopia often results. Hypermetropia is usually under $+3D$ and myopia under $-5D$, i.e. quite thin lenses in spectacles are required. Severe degrees of myopia, with axial lengths up to 35 mm or even greater (occasionally more than $-20D$ of myopia) are more common than severe degrees of hypermetropia (seldom greater than $+8D$).

Presbyopia

There are only three certainties in life: birth, death and presbyopia. The last affects almost the whole white population by their mid-forties, and Asians and Afro-Caribbeans by their mid-thirties, when they become dependent on spectacles for reading. Since 100% of the population will be affected, it is important to understand the mechanism, as follows.

In 'accommodation', the ciliary muscle contracts so that the fibres of the suspensory ligament of the eye lens become less taut, i.e. looser; see Fig. 3.2a. The eye lens then 'indulges its natural tendency to get fatter', i.e. its surfaces become more steeply curved as it becomes rounder, because it is less constrained by the suspensory ligament. Accordingly, the optical power of the eye lens increases. Consider an emmetropic eye, as in Fig. 3.2a or an ametropic eye corrected for distance by spectacles: by definition, parallel rays of light from infinity will be brought to a focus on the retina. When such an eye looks at a near object (Fig. 3.2a) rays of light from that near object will be diverging when they reach the eye. In order to avoid a blurred retinal image of that near object, the eye 'accommodates' very precisely to bring these diverging rays to a focus on the retina (Fig. 3.2a). At the age of 8 years, our maximum power of accommodation is around 14 dioptres, giving a near point of $(^1/_{14} \times 100)$ cm $= 7.1$ cm. That 'near point of distinct vision' gradually recedes throughout life because the eye lens very slowly becomes harder, i.e. less and less able to change shape — *not* because of weakening of the ciliary muscle. When our near point reaches about $^1/_3$ metre, the usual reading distance, we notice that small print is blurred — *the* symptom of presbyopia — and we have to obtain our first 'presbyopic' spectacles (Fig. 3.2b). These usually have a strength of $+0.75D$, or $+0.75D$ is added to our distance correction, if any. But the process of hardening of the eye lens continues so that our near point recedes further and further away. Every 5–7 years the strength of our

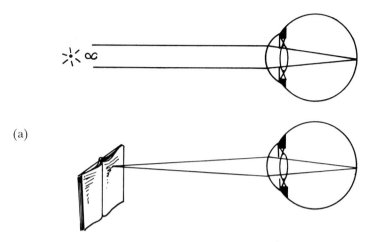

(a)

Fig. 3.2. (a) *Upper*: the emmetropic eye with accommodation completely relaxed brings parallel rays of light from a point source at infinity (∞) to a focus on the retina. *Lower*: the pre-presbyopic emmetropic eye can deal with diverging rays of light from a near object by 'accommodation', i.e. contraction of the ciliary muscle (black part-rectangle) which loosens the suspensory ligament of the lens, which then indulges its natural tendency to get fatter, with more steeply curved (and optically more powerful) surfaces. Print is thus focused on the retina.

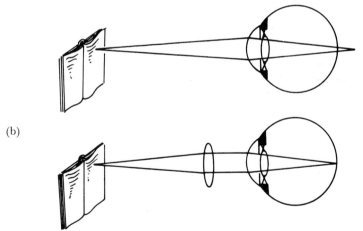

(b)

Fig. 3.2 (b) *Upper*: the presbyopic eye suffers from hardening of the lens, which cannot change shape enough in spite of 'accommodation'. Diverging rays would be brought to a focus behind the retina, i.e. print produces a blurred image on the retina. *Lower*: a biconvex spectacle lens reduces the divergence of the rays enough to allow the eye to bring the rays of light to a focus on the retina. In this example of an eye of an older presbyope (over 65) with no residual accommodation, the spectacle lens has had to be powerful enough to make the diverging rays parallel so that this emmetropic eye can focus the rays on the retina.

'reading addition' has to be increased by +0.5D or +0.75D until around the age of 65 years we have lost all of our accommodation. At that stage a +2.75D addition is required (which is more comfortable than the +3D addition theoretically required for reading at ⅓ m). Any change in refraction after 65 years usually suggests the onset of cataract (nuclear sclerosis imposes myopia), or diabetes (varying levels of intralenticular glucose plus fluid cause varying degrees of swelling of the eye lens with concomitant variations in curvature and *variable* visual acuity).

A stronger reading addition of +4D or +5D or even more may be useful to allow some patients to hold print closer to the eyes than 0.33 m, thereby achieving greater magnification. Base-in prisms are usually incorporated into these lenses in both eyes to relieve the inevitable strain on convergence (p. 38, Fig 4.1). Such spectacles are particularly useful in patients with macular degeneration (p. 112), even in the teenager or young adult, or in early cataract if operation has to be avoided or postponed.

Reading Spectacles

The solution to the problem of presbyopia is very much a matter of individual patient's preference, with guidance from the optometrist or ophthalmologist (see Fig. 3.3). The difficulty arises eventually for everyone whether or not they already have a refractive error requiring distance spectacles. The obvious cure is a separate pair of reading spectacles. But a distant object seen through 'readers' is blurred, so the presbyope has to remove her readers to see a distant object clearly; or, if ametropic, has then to put on her distance spectacles. Frustration ensues. Since she usually looks downwards to read, the emmetrope often chooses half-glasses, looking over their tops to see for distance, or may choose bifocals in which the distance (upper) lens is plain glass. The ametrope would choose *bifocals* in which the distance (upper) part corrects her distance refractive error while the reading part had the 'extra +' addition required to clarify print, etc.

Bifocals were accepted as very satisfactory for many decades. Unfortunately, the 65 + year-old could see clearly only at infinity and at a reading distance of, say, 0.33 m with a +3D reading lens (in practice +2.75D is more comfortable). *Trifocals* were devised to add a chosen intermediate distance — the furthest extent of the entrepreneur's desk top, or the music stand of the musician. However, some found bifocals and trifocals intolerable because of the 'jump' at the transition.

Multifocals are the almost ideal solution to the problem (Fig. 3.3). A method exists for grinding an increasing curvature on the surface of spectacle lenses so that, as her gaze moves downwards, the presbyope

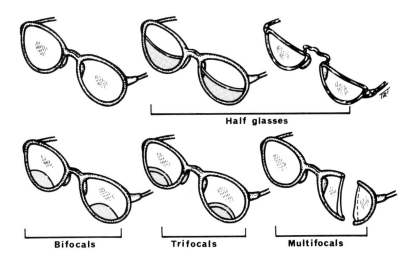

Half glasses

Bifocals   **Trifocals**   **Multifocals**

Fig. 3.3. Spectacles that treat presbyopia, utilizing the fact that reading is usually done with gaze directed downwards. The top left are pure reading spectacles which have to be removed when the patient wants to see clearly in the distance. For the severely presbyopic, clear vision at a distance, or distances, between infinity and reading distance can be obtained with trifocals, or multifocals, respectively.

can see increasingly close objects until, most inferiorly, print at reading distance is clear. This is acceptable to the majority of patients, but they should be warned of 'swimming' in their peripheral fields as their gaze moves downwards. Adaptable patients lose this sensation within a few days or a week, but some cannot cope, and have to fall back on bifocals or separate distance and reading glasses. An advantage of multifocals is that 'wearers' do not demonstrate to the onlooker that they are in the presbyopic age group! Some carry that objective to its logical conclusion and wear a contact lens in one eye to correct it for near vision while the other eye, if emmetropic, has no contact lens or, if ametropic, has a contact lens with a correction for distance! Bifocal contact lenses are also available.

It is important for any general clinician to be able to decide from a patient's spectacles what her refractive error is. The reason is that refractive errors are not just optical problems: see sections on hypermetropia and myopia below. See 'Refraction' later in this chapter for the technique of estimating refractive errors.

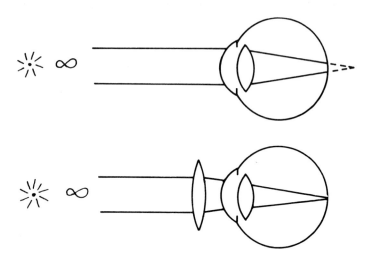

Fig. 3.4. Hypermetropic (US hyperopic) or long-sighted eye. *Upper*: axial length is usually 'too short' for the eye's dioptric power so that, with accommodation relaxed, parallel rays would be brought to a focus behind the retina. *Lower*: an appropriate convex or plus lens 'cures' the condition.

Hypermetropia

Hypermetropia or long-sight (US hyperopia) is applied when parallel rays of light from effective infinity would be brought to a focus behind the retina, accommodation being fully relaxed (Fig. 3.4). The cause is usually an abnormally short axial length of eyeball, not fully compensated by increased curvature of cornea and surfaces of the eye lens. Both eyes are almost invariably affected from birth, usually equally, and heredity is a factor. The eyes can 'cure' this for themselves, except in very severe cases, by exerting accommodation (p. 20): the eyes can often tolerate this extra effort for years but presbyopia will occur at an earlier age than usual. The association between accommodation and convergence (the 'near reflex' includes both) explains the frequency of convergent strabismus in child hypermetropes described in Chapter 4.

A convex (or 'plus' or + lens) of appropriate power will 'cure' this condition (see Fig. 3.4). As the power of accommodation diminishes throughout life, the power of the correcting lens has to be increased. When accommodation has disappeared completely (presbyopia, p. 20), by 65 years, the hypermetrope not only needs convex spectacles for constant use to see clearly in the distance but, of course, requires a reading addition of about + 3D added to the power of that distance lens.

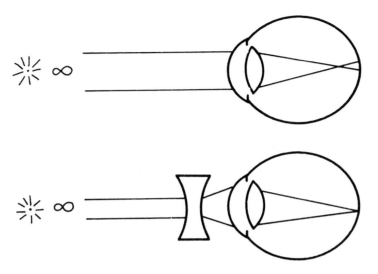

Fig. 3.5. Myopic or short-sighted eye. *Upper*: axial length is usually 'too long' for the eye's dioptric power so that parallel rays are focused in front of the retina. *Lower*: a concave or minus lens 'cures' the condition.

Myopia

Myopia or short-sight means that parallel rays of light from effective infinity are brought to a focus in front of the retina, accommodation being fully relaxed (see Fig. 3.5). The cause is usually a greater than normal axial length of eyeball, not fully compensated by some flattening of the cornea and surfaces of the eye lens (Fig. 3.1). Both eyes are almost invariably affected, usually equally. Unlike hypermetropia, which is usually congenital, myopia usually starts around the age of 7 years in previously emmetropic eyes, and progresses until the middle or late 'teens. Heredity is a factor. Also unlike the hypermetrope, the myope cannot compensate for her optical handicap in distance vision, although she can usually see to read without, or with less, accommodation. A concave spectacle lens, not very strong, will 'cure' most patients (Fig. 3.5). Like everyone else, a myope becomes presbyopic. The usual reading addition to her spectacles will be required for close work: by the age of 65 about + 3D. Note that a + 3D addition completely neutralizes a – 3D myope's distance correction, i.e. her reading 'lens' is plain glass; a – 3D myope will be able to read print at 0.33 m with no accommodation at all.

As in the case of hypermetropia, myopia is associated with certain eye diseases. Most cases of retinal detachment are myopes (over 50%), but the proportion of myopes who develop retinal detachment is not high, around 2–3% albeit much higher than the proportion of emmetropes and hypermetropes. There is a much less strong association with open angle glaucoma and with cataract. The correlation with macular degeneration in the elderly is moderate.

Astigmatism

Astigmatism describes the situation where the curvature of the cornea is not equal in every meridian. This is subdivided into 'regular' and 'irregular' astigmatism (see Fig. 3.6).

Regular Astigmatism
A slight 'buckling' of the cornea is by far the commonest cause of astigmatism: the convexity in one direction is less or greater than in the other at right angles. The road surface of a bicycle tyre demonstrates this very well in an exaggerated form: in the plane of the wheel, the curvature is very much flatter than in any plane at right angles to it. The optical effect can be seen in Fig. 3.6. Note that each point on an object will produce two foci at different distances. Minor degrees are common. Significant regular astigmatism is congenital, bilateral, and uncommon; it is usually discovered first at the vision test taken at entry to school. It may accompany hypermetropia or myopia. A spectacle lens ground with different curvatures at right angles to each other can usually be devised to correct this defect.

Irregular Astigmatism
The surface of the central area of the cornea opposite the pupil may be bumpy, usually with some opacification in the cornea deep to that surface. The commonest cause is probably injury by a sharp object, possibly followed by infection and a corneal ulcer (see. p. 150). Another cause may be a central dendritic ulcer (herpes simplex) with fibrosis on healing (see p. 85). Rays of light meeting the surface are scattered in all directions, aggravated by any opacity in the corneal stroma, hence there is very poor visual acuity. Note that these lesions are usually unilateral.

Corneal dystrophies, by definition *bilateral* and avascular, are rare causes of irregular astigmatism but are very disabling when severe. By far the commonest is keratoconus, which is a gradual bulging outwards of a progressively weak, thinning central cornea. It is usually due to

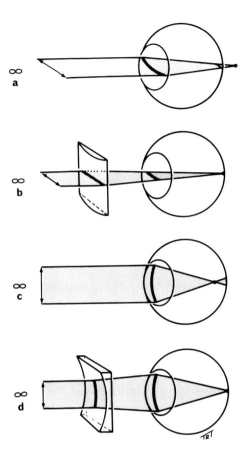

Fig. 3.6. Mixed astigmatism, i.e. one meridian myopic and the other hypermetropic. (a) A broad band of light at right angles to the plane of the paper would be brought to a focus behind the retina. (b) A convex (positive) cylindrical lens converges the rays en route to the eye, which then produces a clear focus in that meridian on the retina. (c) A broad band of light is shown in the plane of the paper; this is brought to a focus in front of the retina. (d) A concave (minus) cylindrical lens diverges the rays en route to the eye, which then produces a clear focus in that meridian on the retina.

A spectacle lens should be prescribed that is concave in one meridian on the front surface and convex in the meridian at right angles to it on the back surface.

autosomal recessive genes. There is a large variety of much more rare corneal dystrophies, usually autosomal dominant, see also p. 121.

Treatment of Refractive Errors

Is any action required? That question is always worth asking in any medical (or other!) situation. For a *unilateral* refractive error or corneal opacity, the authors' answer is usually no. A careful refraction may produce an improvement with a spectacle lens — often not worth the patient's trouble to wear in a unilateral case. We would seldom do a corneal graft in such a case of unilateral irregular astigmatism unless there is a cosmetic handicap, which can well be intolerable to the patient. Even if a spectacle lens fails, improvement of acuity with a pinhole suggests that a contact lens may well succeed (see below); however, if the other eye has good acuity, such patients seldom persevere with a contact lens.

In *bilateral* cases, the situation is of course entirely different. However, refractive errors or keratoconus or other corneal dystrophies are often unequal in the two eyes and a careful refraction can often devise spectacles to overcome enough of the refractive error in the less affected eye to make life tolerable. Sooner or later in keratoconus a contact lens in one or both eyes — the standard treatment — often becomes necessary, and may be followed eventually by a corneal graft. See also p. 121. The operative prognosis in keratoconus is good because the lesion is avascular: the central cornea is 'immunologically privileged', i.e. inaccessible to lymphocytes.

Deprivation Amblyopia

Congenital unilateral hypermetropia, or anisohypermetropia (i.e. greater hypermetropia in one eye than the other), or aniso-astigmatism, often causes a mild form of deprivation amblyopia in the worse eye which can be treated by occlusion until the age of 10 or 12 years, in contrast to strabismic amblyopia which must *not* be treated by occlusion after the age of 6 or 7 years because of the risk of permanent and incurable diplopia. See p. 41 for strabismic amblyopia.

Congenital unilateral cataract will produce a very dense deprivation amblyopia unless operated within the first few weeks (even up to 3 – 4 months) of life *and* corrected with a contact lens or even an intraocular lens. In bilateral cataract, the situation is much less urgent, and operations for both eyes at the age of 6 to 12 months usually suffice.

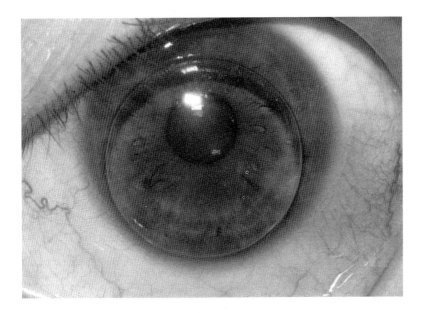

Fig. 3.7. A hard contact lens on the corneal surface moves around freely with movements of the eyeball and blinking, but usually tends to gravitate slightly downwards.

Contact Lenses

Contact lenses are thin, circular lenses that usually lie on the surface of the cornea and correct refractive errors by replacing the anterior surface of the cornea with the anterior surface of the contact lens. See Figs 3.7 and 3.8. (Occasionally, large hard 'scleral haptic' lenses are used: the periphery of these lenses rests on the conjunctiva covering the sclera so that the central optical dome can achieve clearance over a severely astigmatic, especially keratoconic, cornea.) A thin film of tears intervenes between the contact lens and the cornea: all three have very similar refractive indices. The major indication for contact lenses is bilateral irregular astigmatism e.g. keratoconus. Another indication is bilateral high myopia, or high hypermetropia (e.g. aphakia, which means absence of the eye lens, usually following cataract extraction); contact lenses improve the restricted field of vision and distortion imposed by thick spectacle lenses. Most contact lenses, however, are worn for cosmetic reasons in low degrees of myopia. A significant proportion of patients who try contact lenses abandon them after a few

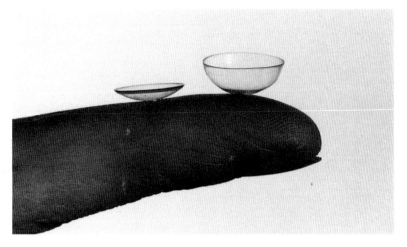

Fig. 3.8. A soft contact lens sits nearer the finger tip; the smaller lens is a hard contact lens.

weeks or months because of discomfort, although in most cases the initial feeling of foreign body quickly diminishes because corneal sensation becomes blunted. The various types can be subdivided into two main groups.

- Hard, rather brittle, contact lenses are made of polymethylmethacrylate (acrylic) and cover most of the cornea, having a diameter of 8 – 10 mm (see Figs 3.7 and 3.8). Their back curve is slightly steeper than that of the cornea, while the curvature of the front surface can be ground to correct the refractive error: less steep than the anterior corneal surface in the case of myopes (p. 25), and steeper in the case of hypermetropes (p. 24). These lenses can be worn for only a few hours at a time because oxygen from the air cannot reach the corneal epithelium: after removal of the lenses for half an hour or so, recovery ensues. Gas-permeable lenses, though 'hard', can generally be worn for longer periods.
- 'Soft' lenses are made of the hydrophilic polymer 'HEMA' (2-hydroxyethylmethacrylate). They are larger than hard lenses and overlap the corneo-scleral junction (limbus). They are more easily tolerated than hard lenses and can be worn for much longer periods.

COMPLICATIONS OF CONTACT LENSES

Careful cleaning and sterilization by chemical solutions (hard lenses) or boiling (soft lenses) are important. Similarly, the containers should be clean and sterile. Corneal ulceration or keratitis (viral, bacterial, fungal or amoebal) is a constant, though small, risk especially in the case of (disposable) extended-wear soft lenses: lenses remaining in situ during sleep overnight increase that risk. Hard, gas-permeable and conventional soft lenses have the lowest risk. Note that water from the tap (and in swimming baths) is a source of acanthamoeba, an occasional culprit in keratitis associated with contact lenses especially if 'rinsed under the tap'. Giant papillary conjunctivitis — like multiple small cobblestones — under both upper and lower lids is one occasional adverse reaction, especially to soft lenses, after some months. Prolonged contact lens wear over a period of years may elicit peripheral but progressive corneal neovascularization. Contact lenses worn for more than 4 years can produce keratoconus in a very small proportion of patients (which is not incompatible with the great value of contact lenses in the management of keratoconus); it may be severe enough to require corneal grafting.

The young and the elderly usually lack the manual dexterity and appreciation of sterility required to cope with contact lenses.

All contact lens wearers should have spectacles available for use if they develop sore eyes. Indeed, the authors recommend that patients minimize their wearing time, and revert to spectacles as often as possible, because of the long-term risks of neovascularization and keratoconus.

Refractive Surgery

In radial keratotomy ('RK') for moderate myopia or astigmatism, about 6–12 very deep incisions are made into the cornea, starting about 2 mm from its centre and radiating out to the corneo-scleral junction; surprisingly, the central area of the cornea flattens. The main long-term complication is glare because of scattering of light rays by the scarred cornea, especially at night when the pupil is dilated. Emmetropia is not always accurately achieved.

Much less invasive is photorefractive keratectomy ('PRK'). Under topical anaesthesia, a very thin layer of central cornea is 'shaved off' by a computer-controlled excimer laser to make the anterior surface of the cornea flatter in myopia. It is much less successful in hypermetropia, in which the corneal surface has to be more steeply curved. Results are more predictable up to $-6D$ than for greater myopia, but precise emmetropia cannot always be obtained. Slight corneal scarring occurs in around 1% of cases under $-6D$ myopia, rising to 9% over $-6D$; a small proportion may lose 1 or 2 lines of visual acuity on Snellen's test chart, and may suffer glare. Occasionally scarring may be severe. Some long-term regression may occur.

In epikeratophakia, a 'lens' made from a donor cornea is sutured to the *surface* of the recipient cornea (compare corneal graft, p. 121); the curvature of the surface of the donor lens alters the recipient's refraction, but its mechanical supportive effect can be utilized in keratoconus (see p. 28 and p. 121).

The management of refractive errors associated with cataract operations and aphakia is described in Chapter 8.

Assessment of Refractive Errors

PINHOLE TEST

A pinhole can be made in a card, or a pinhole disc can be purchased from an optical supplier or an optometrist. If a patient has subnormal visual acuity that improves to (almost) normal when she looks through a pinhole held close to her eye, then that eye suffers only from a refractive error. This test is very useful for general practitioners and physicians, especially neurologists, and casualty officers. The rationale is that the refracting system of the eye is almost eliminated (compare the pinhole camera) because a very narrow bundle of rays of light from each point on the object passes almost through the nodal point of the eye's lens system: rays of light from any direction pass undeviated through the nodal point of any lens system. (The nodal point is usually around the geometrical centre of a lens.)

'REFRACTION'

The student should try to observe this basic skill being practised by opticians (optometrists) or eye specialists, at least on one occasion. This account is merely an outline.

Stage I. Although autorefractometers and refraction technicians are establishing themselves in stage I of this process, a retinoscope (skiascope) is still often employed by the refractionist to assess 'objectively' and quite accurately the degree of a patient's refractive error.

A retinoscope (skiascope) is rather similar to an ophthalmoscope, but merely projects a streak or spot of usually parallel rays of light through the patient's pupil. These rays are reflected back from the fundus of the patient's eye through the patient's pupil and are viewed by the observer through the retinoscope's peephole. From a distance of about 1 m, a spot or streak of light from a retinoscope is shone into one pupil of a patient whose other eye is looking at an infinitely distant object to relax her accommodation. (A child's accommodation has to be paralysed by eye drops of tropicamide, homatropine or, especially in dark brown eyes, atropine).

The refractionist tilts the instrument so that the spot of light on the retina moves up and down, then from side to side. The observer concentrates on the direction of movement of the light emerging from the pupil. If these reflected rays are seen by the observer to move in the *opposite* direction to that of the tilting of the instrument, then the patient is myopic. The reason for the 'opposite' movement is that in a myope (of more than about $-1.0D$), a real image of the spot of light on the fundus is produced between the patient's eye and the observer's eye. The refractionist takes progressively stronger *minus* (concave) lenses from his lens box and inserts them into the trial frame, until the 'opposite' direction of movement is reversed to a 'with' movement. The lens that *just* produces the change-over indicates the degree of myopia of the patient.

If the reflected rays are seen to move in the *same* direction as the movement imposed on the in-going rays by the tilting of the instrument, then the patient is hypermetropic (or emmetropic, i.e. with no refractive error) or very slightly myopic, because the test is conducted by an observer about 1 m from the patient. (If the observer were infinitely far away using a searchlight, a zero lens, i.e. plain glass, would indicate emmetropia!). The reason for the 'with' movement in hypermetropia is that the rays of light emerging from the patient's pupil come from a virtual image behind her retina. The refractionist then finds the minimum plus (convex) lens required to change the direction of movement (a $+1.0D$ lens indicates emmetropia, while a $+0.5D$ lens indicates $-0.5D$ of myopia).

If there is a difference between the lenses required to change the direction of movement in two meridians at right angles to each other, then regular astigmatism is present. The axis of astigmatism may not be vertical or horizontal, but oblique.

Stage II. This is the more subjective part of this investigation and is used for all patients. The refractionist tests each eye separately. She inserts in the trial frame a trial lens based on her retinoscopy (skiascopy) or auto-refraction findings. The patient, sitting 6 m from the test chart, is then asked to read as far down as possible. The refractionist changes the lens to a more or less powerful one and asks the patient if her visual acuity has improved. The lens that provides the best visual acuity is usually the one prescribed. For patients in the presbyopic years, an additional test is done with small print held at the usual reading distance (Fig. 3.2a,b and Fig. 2.2); the distance lens (if any) is modified by $+0.75D$ to $+2.75D$ depending on the addition that makes the print comfortably clear.

A lens prescription can be understood with a little practice. The most easily interpreted format is

$$\text{R} \qquad\qquad \text{L}$$

$$\frac{+2.00}{+2.00\big\downarrow_{90}} = 6/6 \qquad\qquad \frac{+2.00}{+2.00\big\downarrow_{90}} = 6/6$$

which says that each eye has normal visual acuity (6/6) with a spectacle lens consisting of a $+2.00$ dioptre sphere and a $+2.00$ dioptre cylinder with its axis vertical, i.e. 90 degrees. Note how symmetrical the two eyes usually are. Another way of writing this is

$$\text{R} \quad +2.0 \text{ DS}/ +2.0 \text{ DC at } 90 \text{ (6/6)}$$
$$\text{L} \quad +2.0 \text{ DS}/ +2.0 \text{ DC at } 90 \text{ (6/6)}$$

A 'spherical' lens has equal power in all meridians, whilst a 'cylindrical' lens has greater power in a specific meridian. The lens described by the above prescription has a power of $+2$ dioptres (2 dioptre sphere) in one meridian and $+4$ dioptres in another meridian (i.e. $+2$ dioptre sphere with $+2$ dioptre cylinder).

'Diagnosis' of an Unknown Spectacle Lens
This can be done quickly after a little practice. At least the clinician should be able to decide quickly whether an unknown lens is concave, i.e. minus or – (for a myope), or convex, i.e. plus or + (for a hypermetrope or presbyope), and whether a correction for astigmatism is present. Students should ask a member of staff for a practical demonstration, on the following basis.

- Take the patient's spectacles and start with her right lens. You are assumed to be emmetropic or wearing your correct spectacles.
- Hold the lens as close as possible to your own master eye (usually the right) *by turning the ear pieces away from your face.*
- Look through the lens at an object as far away as possible, e.g. out of the window, or at least on the other side of the room. If the object looks smaller (but usually remaining clear) the unknown is a concave (minus or negative) lens; if larger (but usually blurred) the lens is convex (plus or positive).
- A better test is to move the unknown lens up and down and from side to side while looking at a distant object as before. If the object appears to move in the same direction as the movement of the lens under test ('with movement'), it is concave (minus or negative); if the object appears to move in the opposite direction ('against

movement'), the test lens is convex (or plus or positive). No movement indicates plain glass, of course. Do not confuse this description (important for all) with that of retinoscopy in small print under 'Refraction' above (only really important for the specialist).

The reason for the with and against movements is that a minus lens produces a virtual image between the object and the lens, whereas a plus lens would produce a real image behind the observer's eye. A strong minus lens will have an obviously thick edge while a strong plus lens will have a thick centre: feel them with your fingers. To make a more accurate assessment take lenses from a box of trial lenses and neutralize the movement (positive lenses for minus spectacle lenses, and vice versa, of course): the strength of the trial lens indicates the power of the unknown lens. A focimeter can be used for this purpose.

To diagnose astigmatism, take the unknown spectacle lens and hold it about an inch in front of your master eye so that you can see a distant vertical or horizontal line (e.g. a distant building or the corner of the room) simultaneously outside the lens *and* through the lens. If the two lines are not continuous, rotate the unknown lens until they are continuous. Then rotate the lens about 5–10 degrees; if astigmatism is present, the line as seen through the spectacle lens appears to rotate around the centre of the lens (independently of the line as seen outside the lens of course). The strength of any sphere and cylinder can then easily be estimated by neutralization, or by using a focimeter.

UNNECESSARY SPECTACLES

For small degrees of refractive error of any sort, especially if unilateral, the authors do not usually prescribe spectacles. If these are supplied, most patients will soon abandon them. No permanent harm to the eyes accrues from this, or indeed from wearing the wrong spectacles, except in occasional cases in young children.

CHANGES OF SPECTACLES

The authors' policy is to see most patients with spectacles about every 5–7 years, with a few exceptions, e.g. small children (whose frames are understandably often damaged) or in the first years of myopia when it is progressing quickly; in these examples, a re-refraction every 9 months or so may be advisable.

The 5–7 year rule applies even in presbyopia, because an increase in the strength of presbyopic correction of about + 0.75D is the authors' usual practice (starting with a + 0.75D addition at 45 years). The strongest correction for normal eyes is usually a + 2.75D addition at age 65. A patient aged 52 will usually receive + 1.50D addition, after refraction, while a 59-year-old will usually require a + 2.25D addition, which leaves a final correction of a + 2.75D addition at 65 years. Even if the starting lens has only a + 0.5D addition, and each increment is + 0.5D, a re-refraction every 5 years is all that is usually required.

Chapter 4

SQUINT OR STRABISMUS

Divide all your squinting patients as soon as possible into two groups (a) concomitant and (b) incomitant, by testing the ocular movements. These may be easily differentiated: in a 'concomitant' squint, the visual axes maintain the same abnormal angle to one another in all directions of gaze, while in an 'incomitant' squint the angle between the visual axes (i.e. the degree of squint) varies depending upon the direction of looking.

Concomitant squints usually start in childhood, but may well continue into adult life. Incomitant squints usually present in adults with a complaint of diplopia (double vision).

Concomitant Squints

Concomitant Convergent Squint

'Concomitant' is applied when the visual axes maintain the same abnormal angle to each other in all directions of gaze. Most squints in the young children belong to this category, but, even in them, ocular movements must be carefully tested, often in each eye separately (the parent covering up the other eye), to exclude an incomitant squint. Note that urgent referral to an ophthalmologist, say within a week at most, is important to minimize strabismic amblyopia.

Hypermetropia (US: hyperopia) is an important factor in causing concomitant squint. To understand the connection, we must apply some of the considerations of accommodation described on p. 20 to *both* eyes. See Fig. 4.1. In emmetropia (i.e. eyes with no refractive error), when both eyes are used for close work, accommodation occurs in each eye so that a clear image is focused on the macula. To avoid diplopia, the visual axes must be converged on the object of interest, i.e. both medial recti contract simultaneously by an amount closely geared to the amount of accommodation: this is the accommodation – convergence reflex.

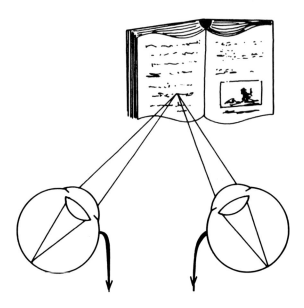

Fig. 4.1. Do not confuse convergence of rays of light and contraction of both medial recti, also called convergence. Convergence, i.e. contraction of *both* medial recti simultaneously, accompanies accommodation for close work (see also Fig. 3.2). Accommodation, i.e. contraction of the ciliary muscle, loosens the suspensory ligament of the lens, and so allows the eye lens to become rounder therefore to have more curved and optically more powerful surfaces. Accommodation is required to converge on the retina diverging rays from a near object. To avoid double vision, *both* medial recti have to contract very precisely to ensure that *both* visual axes are converged on the object of interest, whose images can be sited on the fovea in each eye. The accommodation–convergence reflex is very accurate.

Hypermetropia (p. 24) occurs when the size of the eyeball is smaller than usual, including its axial length. Both eyes are affected equally in the majority of cases. With the two visual axes directed towards infinity (they are of course parallel), *and with accommodation entirely relaxed*, a blurred image would appear on both hypermetrope's retinae; see Fig. 4.2. To clarify even the distant image, these eyes have to accommodate, which in turn is associated with contraction of both medial recti, i.e. convergence (Fig. 4.1). For low degrees of hypermetropia, the brain can inhibit this tendency to converge, so that for distance the visual axes can struggle to remain parallel, at least initially. However, when the

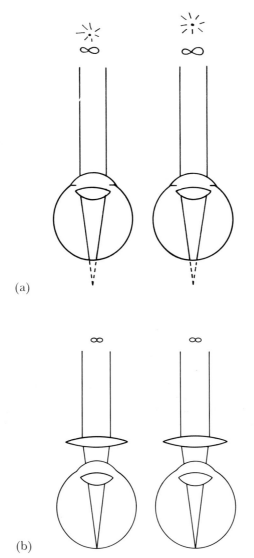

(a)

(b)

Fig. 4.2. (a) Horizontal section through a pair of hypermetropic (long-sighted) eyes looking into the far distance with *accommodation completely relaxed*. Parallel rays of light from infinity (∞) produce blurred images on the retinae. To see clearly *even for distance*, such eyes have to accommodate, which stimulates convergence. If the powerful accommodation – convergence reflex (see Fig. 4.1) cannot be inhibited, a convergent squint ensues even for distance; the situation is even more unstable for a near object. (b) A biconvex spectacle lens in front of each eye 'cures' the hypermetropia by starting to focus the parallel rays before they reach the eye. Convergence is no longer stimulated for distance.

hypermetropic child looks at a near object, more accommodation is added, so more convergence is also stimulated: the accommodation – convergence reflex is very strong in the young, much less so in adults. That unstable situation tends to break down into a convergent squint of one eye — not both eyes simultaneously since the child retains the use of one eye to allow him to see the object of interest clearly. Occasionally an alternating squint develops, i.e. sometimes the right and sometimes the left eye converges. Much more often, only one eye squints. The squinting eye may be more hypermetropic than the other, or have (more) astigmatism, but usually we cannot find a reason for that particular eye to converge. Accordingly this squint tends to be noticed first for near objects, especially when the child is tired, hungry, angry or ill. As shown in Fig. 4.2b, convex (+) spectacle lenses 'cure' the hypermetropia and, if supplied early and urgently, may cure the squint.

The diagnosis is usually obvious, having been made by a relative already. A good clue lies in asymmetry of the corneal reflections — one or two bright spots of light reflected by the anterior corneal surface, which acts as a convex mirror. See Fig. 4.3b and compare Fig. 4.4.

The *cover/uncover test* is very useful in the diagnosis of constant squint especially if it is only slight. See Figs 4.3a to e (pp. 42 and 43). Although it is simple and appears easy, it requires much practice. Attend the orthoptic department to practise on many squinting patients. The patient should be looking at a distant object, say the top letter of the Snellen's test chart. For a young child, however, we must be content with her looking at an interesting picture (Fig. 4.3a) held at about 1 m from her eyes, preferably on the bridge of the examiner's nose. For technique, see the captions to Figs 4.3a to e. (Do *not* try to learn the alternating cover test until you are very experienced.)

Epicanthic folds produce the appearance of a squint, especially in the very young child, before the bridge of the nose develops and takes up the slack (see Figs 4.4 and 12.5). In such cases, symmetry of the corneal reflections and a negative cover/uncover test will help to exclude a constant squint. Visual acuity in each eye must be equal, of course.

As soon as the diagnosis of a concomitant convergent squint has been made, the management is very specifically and urgently in the following order:

1. Refraction to correct with spectacles any underlying hypermetropia and examine the fundi. See p. 32 for the method.

2. Occlusion (patching) of the good eye to correct amblyopia in the squinting eye.
3. Surgical correction of any residual squint after the above treatment. N.B. Surgery is *not* necessary in the majority of patients presenting with a squint.

REFRACTION

As soon as an ophthalmologist sees a child with a convergent squint, he will want to provide spectacles *urgently* to correct the hypermetropia that is usually an important underlying factor. Eye drops of a cycloplegic (see below) are instilled into both eyes — preferably by a parent at home to minimize the child's anxiety.

Atropine 1% may be used (guttae, i.e. eye drops, or oculentum, i.e. an eye ointment), especially for brown-eyed children, but a shorter-acting drug such as homatropine 1% or 2% or cyclopentolate (mydrilate) 1% instilled 2 hours and 1 hour before retinoscopy (see Chapter 3) usually suffices. The main objective is to paralyse the child's accommodation so that the ophthalmologist can assess the full amount of the hypermetropia by skiascopy (retinoscopy). See p. 32 for the method. *Another objective is to allow the ophthalmologist to examine both fundi in some detail to exclude disease (rare) in the transparent media (e.g. cataract, vitreous opacities) or in the retina (e.g. choroiditis, retinoblastoma)*: note that, in a child, an eye blinded by these conditions will produce a concomitant squint but it is usually divergent.

The sooner the child wears spectacles the better. Indeed, ideally and rather theoretically, spectacles to correct fully the hypermetropia should cure that squint, if they are worn as soon as the squint is first noticed. In practice, delay usually prevents such a happy outcome, except in cases of intermittent squint.

STRABISMIC AMBLYOPIA AND OCCLUSION

A child who is merely suspected of squint should be seen by an ophthalmologist within a week at most of its being first noticed. An important reason is that, as soon as a squint starts, the child suppresses the diplopic image from the affected eye, and this strabismic amblyopia quickly progresses in severity until the visual acuity is less than 6/60. Unless treated quickly by occlusion of the normal eye, this unilateral near-blindness can become permanent. After the age of 5 or 6 years occlusion has little or no effect, and beyond the age of about 7 years *occlusion of the good eye should be avoided because it may well produce incurable diplopia with little or no effect on the strabismic amblyopia.*

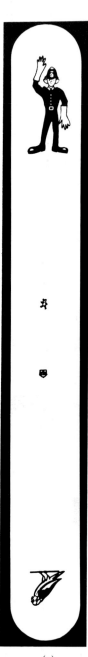

Fig. 4.3. Cover test (a) This tongue-depressor (actual size) is decorated with pictures to interest a 2–6-year-old. She is asked to 'keep looking at the policeman's hat' or 'the little bird's beak'. (Note that an incomitant squint has been excluded by a test of ocular movement *before* the cover test is started.) (b) Even to a lay observer, the right eye obviously has a convergent squint, i.e. the eye is turned inwards towards the nose. The diagnosis is confirmed because the corneal reflection, which is the bright spot of light in the centre of the left pupil, is displaced temporally on the right side. (The corneal surface acts as a convex mirror to reflect an image of light from a window, torch, etc.) (c) The examiner crisply covers the left eye (without touching the face) but watches the right eye, which moves laterally to take up fixation. Therefore, the right eye was converged before the left was covered, i.e. a right convergent squint is diagnosed. When the squint is less marked, the observer must look very carefully for the small movement that allows the eye to take up fixation, and may need to repeat this stage several times. (d) The examiner *uncovers* the left eye, noting the re-convergence of the right eye, and moves the fixation object around to let the eyes return to their usual state. This explains the description 'cover/uncover' test. (e) The examiner crisply covers the right eye and observes that there is no movement in the left, because it is the eye that is consistently maintaining fixation.

(a)

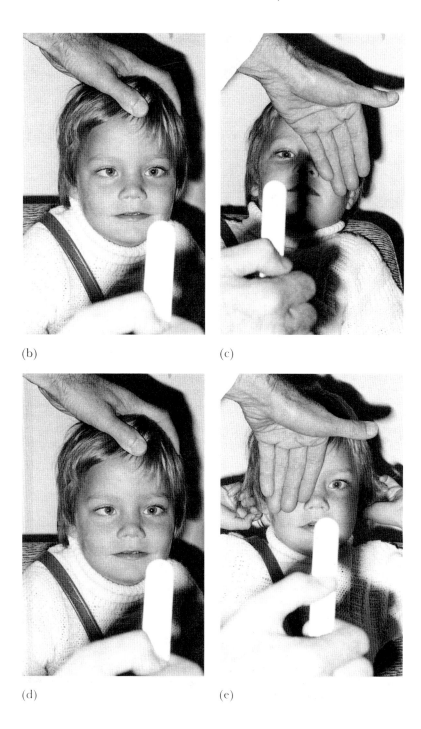

(b)

(c)

(d)

(e)

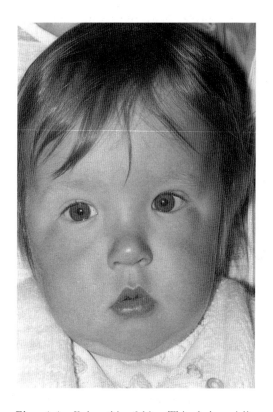

Fig. 4.4. Epicanthic folds. This baby girl's mother was convinced she was 'cross-eyed'. Indeed, at first glance, the observer might conclude that there was a left convergent squint, even allowing that the child is looking slightly to her right. However, closer inspection reveals (a) epicanthic folds, which are crescentic webs of skin obscuring the medial angles (canthi) of the eyelids, and (b) the corneal reflections are precisely symmetrical in relation to the pupils. Cover test is negative. (Of course, a convergent squint may co-exist with, or be added later to, epicanthic folds.) See also Fig. 12.5.

Intermittent occlusion ('patching') of the normal eye under the age of 5 – 6 years will usually reverse strabismic amblyopia, with a fairly rapid increase in visual acuity of the squinting eye. However, it must be realized that occlusion of the normal eye is a specialized technique that must only be undertaken by a ophthalmologist or an orthoptist.

Occlusion must be intermittent, and its duration (and the intervals between) is dependent on the age of the child. *Excessive occlusion of the normal eye, especially in a young child, may result in permanent impairment of vision of the occluded eye (deprivation amblyopia).*

The younger the child, the more quickly amblyopia develops, and the more quickly occlusion will be effective. A week or two in a 18–24-month-old corresponds approximately to 8–10 weeks in a 4-year-old.

It is convenient here to mention deprivation or disuse amblyopia. For example, a child with a congenital *unilateral* cataract must be operated within a few weeks or even 3–4 months of birth, and the eye optically corrected, otherwise that retina will never 'learn' to see. Unilateral severe hypermetropia or unilateral astigmatism (without squint) are other causes.

The 1981 Nobel prize winners, Hubel and Wiesel, have elucidated strabismic and deprivation amblyopia experimentally in kittens and young primates. They produced squint by recession of a medial or lateral rectus muscle plus resection of its antagonist. They produced deprivation in other experiments by tarsorrhaphy (see p. 170). In essence, microelectrodes in the occipital cortex recorded 'silence' from the cortical cells normally activated by the retinal receptors in the squinting or deprived eyes.

SURGERY

Binocular single vision (stereopsis) is lost as soon as a squint in a child becomes permanent. Some ophthalmologists advocate early operation to re-align the visual axes. Recession of one or both medial recti weakens these muscles; in that operation, the insertions are moved posteriorly by about 5 mm. 'Resection' of the lateral rectus muscle or muscles, i.e. excision of 5–8 mm from the anterior end of the muscles, strengthens them. However, full stereopsis is often not retrieved, especially in cases of long-standing squint in an older child. A small degree of residual postoperative convergence due to undercorrection of a convergent squint tends to increase and become obvious within a few weeks or months; a small postoperative divergence due to overcorrection may take years to become obvious cosmetically, or to present because of diplopia, both of which are very difficult to manage. Parents and children should also be warned that the operation cannot correct the underlying refractive error, so that they cannot expect to abandon spectacles postoperatively, much as they would like that outcome. Convergence also tends to diminish with increasing age. All these are reasons why many ophthalmologists prefer to postpone operation until cosmetic considerations become more important, e.g. at the start of school at age 5–6 years or in adolescence.

VALUE OF BINOCULAR SINGLE VISION

How important is full stereopsis? The one-eyed man would tell you he suffers from few handicaps, mainly related to the reduced *field* of vision on the side of the missing eye (e.g. when driving). In the judgement of someone who is totally blind in both eyes, stereopsis must rank as of trivial importance. It is important for aeroplane pilots in the last 100 m of descent, useful for the fast driver, passing another car, who is estimating the spped of head-on approach of another vehicle, and for any surgeon (but there are some excellent one-eyed surgeons!).

Concomitant Divergent Squint

This condition is uncommon. Surprisingly, it is not often associated with myopia. The cause is unknown. It usually presents with an older child or a parent noticing that one eye 'wanders outwards' when looking into the distance or day-dreaming. There is usually no diplopia since a child can suppress the diplopic image. Because the squint is usually intermittent, full binocular vision is retained at most times. But with increasing age, the squint tends to become more frequent (in contrast to concomitant convergent squint, which tends to improve with increasing age) and the possibility of permanent divergence arises. To avoid that, operations are usually done in stages: one lateral rectus muscle is recessed 6–8 mm, then the other, with subsequent medial rectus resection(s) of 5–6 mm over a period of several years.

As mentioned under concomitant convergent squint above, the ophthalmologist will do a refraction (retinoscopy, p. 32 and p. 33) and examine both fundi carefully through a dilated pupil to exclude intraocular disease, especially if the visual acuity is reduced or the child is young.

Diplopia seldom occurs in concomitant convergent squint and is intermittent in concomitant divergent squint. In contrast, *the* presenting feature of *incomitant* squint is double vision.

Incomitant Squints

In incomitant squint, the angle between the visual axes varies according to the direction of looking, i.e. the squint increases in certain directions and decreases in others.

An example will make the term 'incomitant' clear. Suppose the patient has a complete paralysis of the left lateral rectus muscle (see Fig. 4.5.) He will have horizontal diplopia only when he looks to the left, but will have no diplopia in any other direction of gaze. The clinician will observe that when the patient tries to look left, his left eye stops in the straight-ahead position but the right eye moves normally towards the nose. In other words, both the visual axes point to the object of attention in all directions except to the left, i.e. the visual axes do not 'accompany' each other in all directions, hence 'incomitant'. Ask the patient to look at the tip of your forefinger: as you move it to his right and left, then up and down then into the intermediate positions, watch that the eyes move equally in unison except, in this case, to the left.

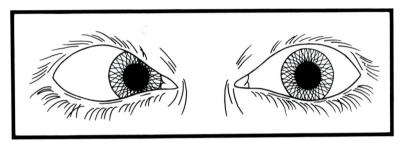

Fig. 4.5. Left lateral rectus (LR) palsy. The patient has been looking at the tip of the examiner's finger, which has been moved to the patient's left at eye level. The left eye has stopped in the 'straight ahead' position whereas the right eye has moved normally, and no symptoms or signs are detectable looking up, down or to the right.

In practice, the presenting symptom in an adult of fairly recent diplopia that *disappears on shutting either eye*, tells you that an incomitant squint is present even though you can detect no abnormality in ocular movements. Children rarely have incomitant squint but it should be excluded in every case: find an interesting toy, or use a flashing light to attract his attention in all directions of gaze — the parent may manage to hold his head reasonably still. It is often necessary to test the ocular movements of each eye separately (covering the other), especially in a child.

A right abducent (VIth) nerve lesion will produce horizontal diplopia to the right. A trochlear (IVth) nerve lesion weakens or paralyses the superior oblique muscle and causes vertical diplopia with a tilt of the image from the squinting eye; the affected eye is unable to move downwards and inwards, essential for reading (see Fig. 4.6).

A complete oculomotor (IIIrd) nerve paralysis does not produce diplopia because ptosis is present! When that drooping upper lid is

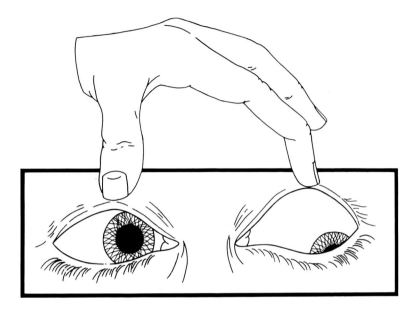

Fig. 4.6. Right superior oblique (SO) palsy. The patient is asked to look at an object down and to his left. The adducted right eye fails to be depressed, with vertical diplopia. (The other action of the SO is to wheel-rotate the 12 o'clock position of the iris inwards, so that a SO paresis adds a tilt to the vertical separation of the diplopic image.) Note that the observer has to hold the patient's upper eyelids up in order to watch movements of the eyes when they look downwards.

lifted, the patient notices double vision, and the eyeball can be seen gazing laterally because of the unopposed action of the intact lateral rectus muscle (VIth nerve); the eyeball is unable to move from that position in any direction except for a wheel-rotation inwards of 12 o'clock on the iris as a result of the action of the superior oblique muscle, which is the only other extraocular muscle with an intact nerve supply (IVth nerve).

However, these proximate causes of diplopia do not constitute diagnoses. Although many cases will be referred for a neurological opinion, the ophthalmologist often has a contribution to make.

- Diabetes mellitus, systemic hypertension and atherosclerosis are the commonest causes of IIIrd, IVth and VIth nerve palsies, probably owing to disruption of the microvascular blood supply to the nerves. The palsy usually recovers spontaneously within a few weeks.

- Concussion or fractured skull is another common cause of IVth nerve palsy.
- Is there a space-occupying lesion in the orbit (usually with proptosis) or lids which is mechanically interfering with ocular movements?
- Dysthyroid orbital disease or, much less commonly, an enlarged lacrimal gland may be the answer.
- A quite common cause of diplopia seen by the ophthalmologist in an adult is the breaking down of a congenital paresis of an extraocular muscle, usually a superior oblique, hence vertical diplopia.
- Another important cause of horizontal or vertical diplopia lasting a few weeks is multiple sclerosis, involving the abducent (VIth) or trochlear (IVth) nerve respectively.
- Finally the systematic clinician should consider each anatomical point from the muscles (dystrophies, however, rarely produce diplopia) backwards to the brain, starting with the motor end-plate (?myasthenia gravis), then the nerve in the orbit and intracranially, then within the brain.

Do not fall into the trap of searching for an extraocular muscle paresis when a complaint of diplopia is due to *uniocular* disease. This may be a presenting symptom of early cataract in the elderly but should be considered also in a young patient, e.g. with corneal opacity or astigmatism. *That mistake can be avoided if you remember always to ask the patient early in the consultation 'Does the double vision remain if you shut the left eye?' and '. . . right eye?'.*

Gaze Palsies

Patients with gaze palsies are very rare and are seen by neurologists rather than ophthalmologists, because the eye lesion is only a part of a larger disability, often produced by a cerebral thrombosis. A lesion of any part of the cortico-nuclear tracts will interfere with the 'orders' being sent by the cerebral cortex to the IIIrd, IVth and VIth cranial nerve nuclei. For example, a patient may be unable to look to his left because stimuli fail to reach the *left* VIth nucleus *and* that part of the *right* IIIrd nucleus concerned, respectively, with turning the left eye to the left and the right eye to the left (but leaving convergence intact). Diplopia is *not* a feature of a gaze palsy.

Nystagmus

The ophthalmologist would say that the commonest cause of this constant 'wobbling' movement of the eyes is *congenitally* poor vision in both eyes from any cause, e.g. congenital cataract, aniridia. Occasional cases, often quite mild, are due to some unknown lesion in the CNS, often hereditary (X-linked recessive, or, quite remarkably, X-linked dominant). Albinos usually have nystagmus, which may be associated with the extraordinary fact that the proportion of optic nerve fibres that cross at the chiasma is greater than normal, as in Siamese cats.

For the neurologist, the commonest cause of nystagmus is multiple sclerosis (MS). Ask the patient to watch your finger as you move it far to his right (face and head being maintained in the 'straight ahead' position). As he strives to maintain fixation on your finger, you will see his eyes drift towards the centre, then jerk quickly back to fixation. 'Nystagmus to the right' indicates that the jerk is to the right. Laevoversion will usually produce a similar result but it may be more or less marked. Normal eyes will maintain steady fixation.

The railway traveller, and the child being whirled around in play, suffer from physiological nystagmus: a relatively slow movement to retain fixation on an object in the environment is followed by a quick jerk to transfer to a new one when the first is about to disappear.

Chapter 5

GLAUCOMA

Glaucoma is a common problem for patients and eye specialists: 'glaucoma clinics' are often held in eye departments. Its frequency as a cause of blindness could be reduced if not eliminated by earlier diagnosis and treatment: these are emphasized in this chapter. The term is used rather loosely to mean an abnormally high intraocular pressure, but see the definition below. The cause is always a reduced outflow of aqueous humour compared with the inflow, which is a secretion from the epithelium of the ciliary body: see the section on classification later.

Definition

The term glaucoma is applied when an eye has an abnormally high intraocular pressure (IOP); it usually also has a pathological optic disc and loss of field of vision. 'Ocular hypertension' may be applied when only high pressure is present. A level of 16 mmHg is regarded as the mean normal pressure but, like blood pressure, the level varies quite widely between individuals even of the same age and sex, and at different times in 24 hours. The standard deviation (SD) is 2.6 mmHg. A strict 'upper limit of normal' would be 21 mmHg (16 mmHg + 2SD = 21.2 mmHg) and a less stringent limit 24 mmHg (16 mmHg + 3SD = 23.8 mmHg); 24 mmHg or above would be agreed by most as definitely pathological, i.e. as a level at which the field of vision will be affected. (In any 'normal' or Gaussian distribution the mean ±2SD includes 95% of the observations and the mean ±3SD includes more than 99%.) A small proportion of patients have, paradoxically, 'low-tension' or 'normal-pressure' glaucoma with slowly progressive field loss and pathological cupping but no rise in pressure (see p. 72).

Pathophysiology

The eyeball has to be filled with tranparent material. The vitreous gel occupies most of the larger cavity behind the 'iris–lens diaphragm' but aqueous humour fills the anterior chamber and some other places. Aqueous humour, with a composition very like that of cerebrospinal fluid (CSF), is secreted by the ciliary epithelium. See Fig. 5.1 and Fig. 1.1. A little diffuses into the vitreous gel and the lens, but almost all passes forwards round the lens through the fibres of its suspensory ligament, and then through the pupil into the anterior chamber. It escapes from the angle of the anterior chamber through the trabecular meshwork into the canal of Schlemm. See Figs 5.1 and 5.2. The main resistance to the outflow of aqueous is at the endothelium, which is the last layer of the trabecular meshwork before aqueous enters the canal. Endothelial cells engulf droplets of aqueous from the anterior chamber side and 'excrete' them into the canal, probably with a very transient period of through-and-through free passage. Arachnoid villi probably function similarly in relation to CSF.

From the canal of Schlemm, about 10–12 'collector channels' carry the aqueous through the anterior sclera to become clear 'aqueous veins'

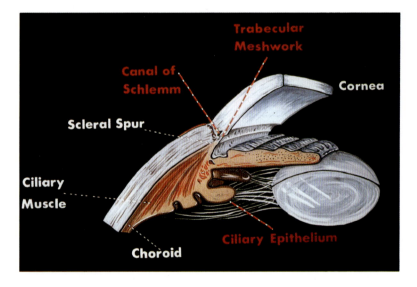

Fig. 5.1. Solid wedge of anterior segment. Main circulation of aqueous humour is lettered in red: secreted by *ciliary epithelium*, it trickles round the eye lens through the suspensory ligament and thence through the pupil into the anterior chamber to escape through the *trabecular meshwork* into the *canal of Schlemm* (see also Fig. 5.2). From there, collector channels carry it to the subconjunctival veins. The ciliary muscle is inserted into the scleral spur and trabecular meshwork: when it contracts (e.g. after pilocarpine) the outflow of aqueous increases. The anterior end of the choroid is just included.

that join ordinary blood-carrying subconjunctival veins. By very careful examination through the slit lamp microscope, these two veins can be seen; for a short distance after they join, there is a 'White Nile' and a 'Blue Nile'.

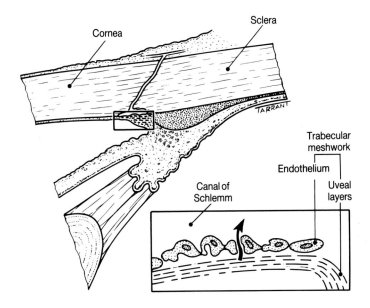

Fig. 5.2. Drainage of aqueous humour. Diagrammatic cross-section at 12 o'clock of the angle of the anterior chamber. The eyeball is looking to the reader's left so that the base of the iris is to the right, cornea to the left and the canal of Schlemm above. The uveal layers of the trabecular meshwork merely filter off, pigment, occasional red blood cells, etc. The main site of resistance to aqueous outflow is the single endothelial layer (see inset). Each cell goes through a cycle of 'ingesting' a droplet of aqueous from the anterior chamber (second and third cell from left), then 'excreting' it into the canal (cell transfixed by arrow and the one on its right). The arrow shows a transient phase of through-and-through drainage. A collector channel is shown leading from the canal of Schlemm to a subconjunctival vein. (Cerebro-spinal fluid is excreted similarly through arachnoid villi.)

About 10% of aqueous in human eyes escapes through 'unconventional channels' by seeping between the cells of the ciliary body exposed in the angle of the anterior chamber at the base of the iris and then between the fibres of the overlying sclera.

The rate of 'aqueous flow' is about 2–3 microlitres (μl) per minute.

All glaucomas are due to defects in outflow of aqueous, none to hypersecretion. Unfortunately, no significant feedback mechanism exists between outflow and secretion.

The end result of greatest concern in glaucoma of any sort is pathological cupping of the optic disc, a special type of optic atrophy, and field loss. See Fig. 5.3a and b. The disc is the softest part of the otherwise resistant corneo-scleral envelope and at pressures above about 24 mmHg the physiological cup enlarges slowly to occupy eventually the whole disc, which is also pushed backwards to become saucerized and pathologically cupped (see p. 73). (The physiological cup is a central area of the optic disc not required for transmission of axons of retinal ganglion cells to the optic nerve. These axons occupy the periphery of the optic disc. The physiological cup may be entirely absent in a small, usually hypermetropic, eyeball or larger than average in a large, usually myopic, eyeball.) In very severe cases, the excavation of the anterior optic nerve extends outwards behind the disc edge to produce an overhang: ophthalmoscopically, the retinal vessels at the disc can be seen to disappear behind the overhang, then to climb out round the disc edge. These effects may be merely the direct result of mechanical pressure, or mediated through interference with the disc's blood supply, or both. That may be an oversimplification because in 'low-tension' or 'normal pressure' glaucoma, pathological cupping is found without raised pressure. These pathognomic disc changes are accompanied by a very characteristic pattern of field loss in all the glaucomas: both will be discussed in more detail in subsequent sections.

Classification of the glaucomas

For most purposes the glaucomas are classified on an aetiological basis as follows. In each case there is a different cause for the obstruction to the outflow of aqueous humour at the angle of the anterior chamber.

Fig. 5.3. The right optic disc (a) has a vertical cup-to-disc (C/D) ratio of about 0.75, i.e. probably pathologically cupped. The cup is the yellowish white oval, long axis vertical, in the centre of the optic disc; the latter has rather indistinct margins. Early glaucomatous field loss (Fig. 5.15) is present and the ocular tension is 24 mmHg. The left C/D ratio is about 0.66 (b). The irregular arc of pigmentation at the temporal edge of the left disc is common and physiological. No glaucomatous field loss is present and the pressure is 22 mmHg. Both angles are open all round on gonioscopy. The inequality between right and left C/D ratios supports the diagnosis of glaucoma.

① DVa 20/OD (Right) / OS (~~Right~~ Left)   Pinhole

② Pupils   Dim Bright
          6.0 → 3.5   ± APD
  Marcus Gunn 6.0 → 3.5

③ VF Confrontations

④ Motility Ductions - Ay itself
           Vergences - Together

External → Symmetry, if Assymetry why

⑤ SLE.
L/L - Lids/Lashes   AC - Anterior chamber
Cy/sclera-   Iris -
K - cornea   Lens -

⑥ DFE | Any Red Top will Dilate
   Vitreous | 2.5% Phenylephrine ⟩ good cocktail
  Optic Nerve Head | 1% Tropicamide
  Macula |
  Vessels | Cyclogyl → last 48%
  Periphery | Atropine 1% → last 1-2 weeks.

MARTIN ARMY COMMUNITY HOSPITAL
MULTIPLE PRESCRIPTION FORM

(Print patient's name)

(Address)   (City)   (State)

(Phone Number)   (Date of Birth)

(Family Member Prefix & Sponsor's SSAN)

Do NOT intermingle regular drugs & Controlled Substances on the same form

Do NOT use form for more than one Controlled Substance

(For Pharmacy Use Only)

(For Pharmacy Use Only)

(For Pharmacy Use Only)

RPh Initials & Notes

MEDICATION	STRENGTH	QUANTITY	DIRECTIONS	REFILLS

Clinic/Service	UCA Code	Date

Prescriber's Signature

Printed/Stamped Name
Rank/Branch/Degree
SSAN

FB (MED) Form 430 (Rev) 1 DEC 83

☆U.S. GOVERNMENT PRINTING OFFICE: 1984 — 750-259/996

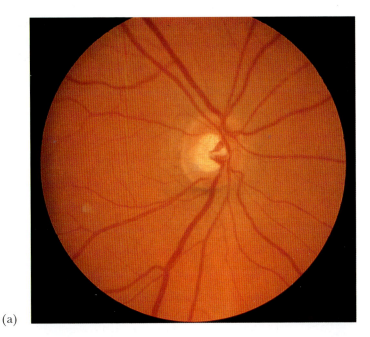

(a)

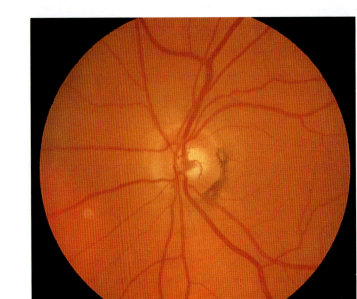

(b)

1. Congenital or infantile glaucoma (buphthalmos)
2. Closed-angle (angle-closure) glaucoma
3. Open-angle (chronic simple) glaucoma
4. Glaucoma due to iridocyclitis, swollen lens, neovascularization, etc., often called 'secondary' glaucoma

(2) and (3), and sometimes (1), are unfortunately often called 'primary' glaucoma. These have an important hereditary basis, especially the first, and a great deal is known about their aetiology.

Details are presented on pp. 65 to 78.

Special Methods of Examination

Students should see these in use in ophthalmic outpatient departments.

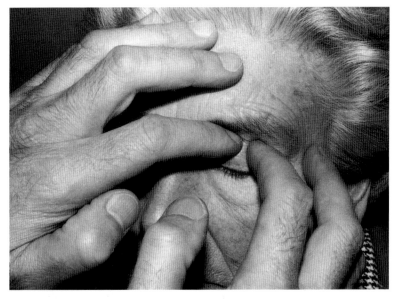

Fig. 5.4. Digital tonometry. The patient is asked to look downwards. The tonometrist places his right and left index fingers on the eyelid over the eyeball, steadying his hands by placing the remaining fingers on the patient's forehead and temple. The right and left index fingers are alternately *gently* depressed into the eyeball to assess 'hard', 'soft' or 'normal'. Compare fluctuation of a cyst or abscess.

TONOMETRY

Since we cannot insert a needle into the human anterior chamber to measure the true intraocular pressure, we must estimate it indirectly by measuring 'ocular tension'. However, the two terms are used interchangeably in practice. Patients experience only minor discomfort from any method because topical anaesthesia is so effective.

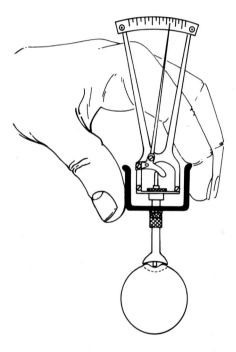

Fig. 5.5. A Schiøtz tonometer is held by the tonometrist so that the footplate rests on the anaesthetized cornea, with only minor discomfort. The lower end of the plunger, emerging from the footplate, indents the cornea — deeply if the intraocular pressure is low (as shown), very little if the IOP is high. The upper end of the plunger transmits the depth of indentation to a lever which in turn moves a long pointer to magnify the indentation. The tip of the pointer moves just in front of a scale in arbitrary units at the top of the picture. The end-point is recorded in arbitrary units but these may be converted by a calibration curve into mmHg.

(a) *Digital tonometry* is the simplest method but is seldom applicable because it will differentiate only rock-hard and soft eyes from the normal. It employs 'fluctuation', which is also applied to cysts, abscesses, etc. See Fig. 5.4.

(b) *Schiøtz tonometry* is not used routinely in many clinics nowadays, because some inaccuracy arises from the unavoidable increase in IOP produced when the instrument is applied to the (anaesthetized) eye. A calibration curve converts scale readings into mmHg. See Fig. 5.5.

(c) Applanation tonometry is very accurate and is the method of choice at present for most ophthalmologists. See Figs 5.6, 5.7 and 5.8. It measures the force required to flatten a standard (small) area of (anaesthetized) cornea. The technique and its explanation follow.

- After a topical anaesthetic, a drop of fluorescein is instilled into the conjunctival sac.

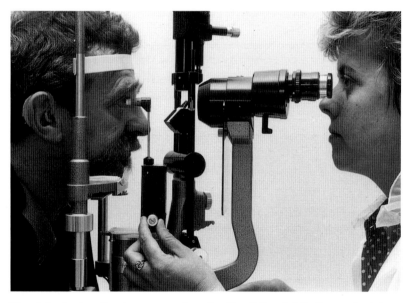

Fig. 5.6. Applanation tonometry. See also Figs 5.7 and 5.8. One end of the applanation 'prism' is in contact with the patient's anaesthetized cornea. Note that it is carried at the top of a stalk based on a 'black box'. The tonometrist has a magnified view through the eyepieces of the slit-lamp microscope of the flat front end of the prism. The force on the prism required to flatten a standard small area of cornea is controlled by the tonometrist's fingers on the milled knob, which transmits that force through a spring-loaded device in the black box to the stalk.

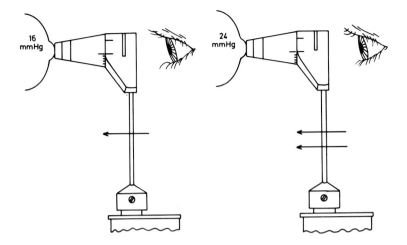

Fig. 5.7. Applanation tonometry. See also Figs 5.6 and 5.8. When the intraocular pressure is 'normal' (16 mmHg) a certain amount of force (←) has to be applied to the applanation 'prism' to flatten a standard area of cornea. That area can be estimated easily by the tonometrist. When the IOP has reached the glaucoma range (24 mmHg and above), a greater force (⇆) is required to flatten the standard area. The force (in grams, which multiplied by 10 gives mmHg) is read off a scale on the milled knob with which the tonometrist controls that force. The instrument is accurate to 1–2 mmHg.

- The plastic 'applanation prism' intervenes between the patient's cornea and the eyepieces of the slit lamp microscope. It is held there at the top of a thin but rigid metal stalk.
- The microscope allows the observer to obtain a magnified view of the plane of the flat front surface of the applanation prism.
- A variable force can be applied to the patient's cornea at the flat applanating surface via the stalk by a milled knob controlled by the observer.
- The end-point, when a standard area of cornea has been 'cleared' of fluorescein, can easily be estimated through the microscope — the applanation prism has a doubling device that separates the upper and lower halves of the ring of fluorescein solution at the edge of the cleared area. See Fig. 5.8.
- When the two half-rings almost overlap, the observer takes a reading from the milled knob, representing a force in grams; that figure × 10 is the value in mmHg.

A hand-held version of this tonometer exists.

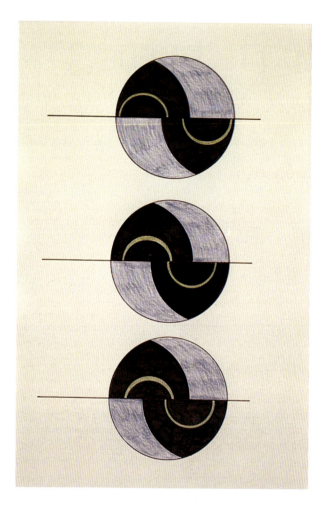

Fig. 5.8. Applanation tonometry. See also Figs 5.6 and 5.7. Observer's view through the eyepieces of the slit-lamp microscope. Fluorescein eye drops have been instilled after a topical anaesthetic. The flat end of the applanation prism flattens a standard area of cornea, which is cleared of fluorescein. The fluorescein forms a complete ring of meniscus around that standard area. A doubling device in the prism converts the ring as seen by the observer into two half-rings. When the force produces the appearance shown in the central diagram, i.e. half-rings not quite overlapping, the reading of pressure is taken. The upper diagram shows the effect of too much force and the lower the effect of too little.

Other tonometers are in use. Optometrists usually prefer a non-contact or puff tonometer, which measures the time taken for a standard jet of air to flatten a small area of the cornea (the end-point being determined by the reflection of a beam of light from the instrument). A pneumatonograph supplies a printout on calibrated paper of ocular tension assessed by the air-pressure on a small floating plastic head required to flatten a standard area of cornea.

GONIOSCOPY

The ophthalmologist must examine the angle of the anterior chamber (gonioscopy, Fig. 5.9) in every patient with raised IOP or suspected of glaucoma. Unfortunately, rays of light emanating from the angle of the anterior chamber are totally internally reflected at the interface between the anterior corneal surface and air (Fig. 5.10). To render these rays

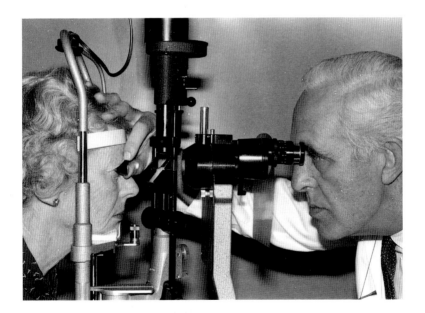

Fig. 5.9. Gonioscopy. See also Fig. 5.10. The patient has a gonioscope applied to her right eye following topical anaesthetic eye drops. The observer sees a magnified view of the angle of the anterior chamber through the eyepieces of the slit-lamp microscope. A gonioscope is fundamentally a contact lens with a curvature steeper than that of the cornea; its bulk is due to a mirror incorporated to reflect rays of light forward into the objective of the microscope.

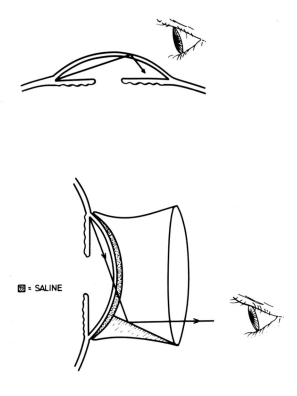

Fig. 5.10. Gonioscope. See also Fig. 5.9. *Upper*: rays of light from the angle of the anterior chamber are totally internally reflected at the air–cornea interface because of the obliquity of the angle of incidence. *Lower*: These rays can now escape because the contact lens of the gonioscope has a steeper curvature than the cornea (saline intervening: the refractive index of cornea, saline and contact lens are very similar). The mirror directs rays of light forwards into the microscope, which magnifies the image for the observer.

visible, the observer applies a contact lens to the surface of the patient's cornea. The layer of saline or tears between the posterior surface of the contact lens and anterior surface of the cornea eliminates the optical effect of the latter since the refractive indices of contact lens, tears and cornea are almost the same. The new surface between air and the contact lens is made steep enough to allow rays to escape (Fig. 5.10). The gonioscope in common use is much bulkier than a contact lens because a mirror is incorporated to reflect rays of light forwards —

merely for convenience — into the microscope through which the observer sees a magnified image of the angle.

FIELDS OF VISION

It is easy to exaggerate the importance of visual acuity, which is a function of a very small area of the central retina (macula and fovea). But we are very dependent on our peripheral fields. Contrast the disability of the patient who suffers from a small bilateral central scotoma that prevents reading or the recognition of faces (most commonly due to macular degeneration) with the handicap of the patient who has lost all his peripheral fields but retains only central vision (most commonly due to open angle glaucoma but also to advanced retinitis pigmentosa; p. 198); although the latter can read with his 'tunnel vision', he cannot cross roads or walk about easily, which the patient with a central scotoma can do. Accordingly, testing and recording of fields of vision are important. The methods are described below.

Confrontation
This is the simplest test but is too gross to detect any but the most advanced case of glaucoma, although it is useful in neurology. The patient and examiner should both be seated, the latter preferably in front of a dark background. See Fig. 2.3 and p. 8. Ask the patient to cover her left eye and to look at your left eye with her right. (The observer shuts his right eye.) In *the middle of each quadrant* of her field (upper and lower temporal, and upper and lower nasal), randomly flutter two fingers noiselessly in a plane midway between patient and examiner, and ask her to 'point to the fingers that are moving'. Examine the left field similarly. Thus hemianopia, a quadrant defect or gross generalized constriction can be detected. *Avoid* testing in the vertical and horizontal meridians: if you test there, a patient with a quadrantanopia or a hemianopia will respond positively even when she sees only half the fingers. 'Inattention defects' can be found by presenting a second pair of simultaneously fluttering fingers on the opposite side of the vertical meridian and again asking the patient to 'point to the fingers that are moving': she will point only to the ones in the more attentive field. See also p. 8.

More precision can be achieved, with, say, a white-headed hat pin. You can demonstrate this by plotting your own blind spot with a small piece of white paper about 1 cm in diameter in a paper clip. Shut your left eye. Look fixedly at a point on the wall 1–2 m in front of you. Hold the paper clip in front of you, at a comfortable arm's length so that the white paper is just to the right of the fixated point. Move the paper horizontally to the right slowly but keep on looking at the fixation point. The paper will disappear less than half a metre from fixation. Note the size of the blind spot by moving the paper in and out of the (physiological) scotoma.

More precise methods are usually required, particularly in cases of glaucoma (see below). They should be seen in use in the outpatient department.

Bjerrum ('Tangent') Screen
A black screen, 1 or 2 m square, is attached to a wall and is evenly illuminated. The patient sits 1 or 2 m respectively from the screen, and shuts her left eye. The right eye looks fixedly at a small white dot in the centre of this black screen. The observer stands well to the side and moves a small white object on the end of a long matt black stick systematically in all areas of the field. Areas in which the patient is not aware of the observer's white spot — scotomas (= blind areas) — are plotted on a chart marked so as to correspond with markings on the Bjerrum screen. The examiner first plots the blind spot, which shows the patient what a scotoma is and checks that she is a good subject, as the vast majority are. The left eye is then examined similarly.

This tangent screen technique provides a magnified plot of quite a large area of the *central* fields (to about 25–30 degrees from fixation) but cannot assess the more peripheral fields.

Goldman Perimeter
A concave bowl (see Fig. 5.11) allows the peripheral field to be plotted as well as the central field. Although the greater magnification of the central field of the 2 m Bjerrum tangent screen (described above) is lost, the precision of Goldman perimetry compensates very well. A spot of light of variable size and intensity is moved systematically around the bowl while the patient fixates a central spot. A semi-automatic plotting device improves efficiency.

Static Perimetry
The methods described above are 'kinetic' methods, depending on *movement* of the test object. In 'static' systems, various random points on a screen or bowl are successively illuminated, at first at subthreshold levels; the intensity is increased until the patient signals that she sees it.

Automated Perimetry
A predetermined programme of static light stimuli is presented to the patient at various points in the visual field, permitting standardization

of visual field assessment and objective recording of the results on a computer data file. Early detection of visual field deterioration in glaucoma is facilitated by increased objectivity in perimetry.

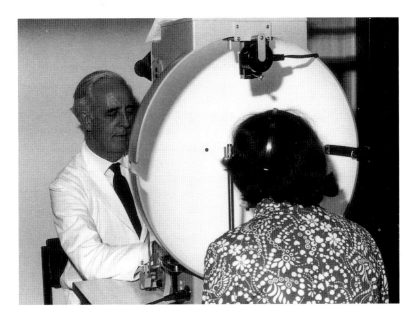

Fig. 5.11. Field plotting on the Goldman perimeter. The patient's right eye is occluded. Her head is on a chin rest. Her left eye maintains fixation constantly on the black spot in the middle of the white bowl. A spot of light is projected (from the lower end of the mobile broad black tube on the patient's right) on to the periphery of the bowl and is moved inwards towards the centre by the perimetrist until the patient signals that she sees it; that point indicates the periphery of the field in that meridian and is recorded semi-automatically. The spot's movement is continued to the centre so that any scotomas (blind spots) can be recorded. The process is repeated in at least a dozen meridians so as to survey the whole field.

Clinical Features, Aetiology and Management

Congenital or Infantile Glaucoma (Buphthalmos)

Cause
In intrauterine life the anterior chamber is filled with tissue originating from the neural crest that has disappeared normally by birth. In rare cases, because of autosomal recessive genes (but males are affected more

often than females), there is persistence of abnormal tissue so that the angle is blocked all round; see p. 202.

Presenting Symptoms

The IOP rises quickly in both eyes, which causes severe pain and photophobia. A constantly crying baby with eyes tightly shut is the result: that combination dictates immediate referral to an ophthalmic surgeon, even if the diagnosis turns out to be acute conjunctivitis or bilateral dendritic ulcers (due to herpes simplex virus).

In response to the rise in pressure, the eyeball of a child under about 2.5 years can enlarge, quite unlike an adult's, hence the term buphthalmos (Greek: ox-eye). Splits in Descemet's membrane, one of the deepest layers of the cornea, are typical: tramlines, about 0.5 mm apart, run irregularly across most of the cornea; they are oedematous because some aqueous has penetrated into the cornea through the splits.

Treatment

Urgent goniotomy under general anaesthesia is required. A knife needle is slid across the anterior chamber, under gonioscopic and microscopic control, to incise the residual tissue in the one-quarter or one-third of the circumference opposite the entry point. A repeat operation for a second one-third may well be required. The prognosis is reasonably good in early cases. Later cases with an opaque enlarged cornea require trabeculectomy or trabeculotomy (see Fig. 5.16) followed by corneal grafting if the pressure can be controlled; blindness is the frequent end-result in late cases. The parents should be warned of the 1-in-8 risk to future siblings (not 1-in-4 for some unknown reason, although the condition is due to autosomal recessive genes).

Closed-angle or Angle-closure Glaucoma (CAG or ACG)

Mechanism

See Figs 5.12, 5.13 and 5.14. Patients predisposed to this disease inherit an eyeball slightly smaller than normal which is often therefore hypermetropic (see Chapters 3 and 4). Around 5% of first-degree relatives will be affected in later life. In an attempt to compensate optically for the short axial length, Nature contrives a lens in the eye which is axially thicker than usual and so has steeper curvatures and is optically more powerful; for the same reason presumably, the lens is placed more anteriorly in this sort of eyeball than usual.

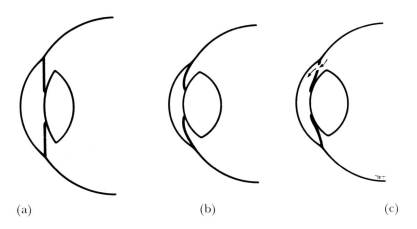

(a)   (b)   (c)

Fig. 5.12. Anterior segments of eyeballs in cross section. (a) An eye with open angle glaucoma and a deep anterior chamber: the iris is all on one plane. (b) The eyeball is predisposed to closed-angle glaucoma. It is smaller overall than (a), has a smaller-diameter cornea and an axially thicker lens placed more anteriorly, hence a shallower anterior chamber and a narrow angle. *Accordingly, aqueous humour meets resistance at the pupil hence ballooning of the iris (iris bombé)*, which narrows the angle even more. The lens goes on growing in size throughout life, aggravating the relative pupil block and causing the anterior chamber to become even more shallow until the peripheral iris closes off the trabecular meshwork (often suddenly to produce acute closed-angle glaucoma). (c) A prophylactic peripheral iridectomy before the angle closes allows aqueous humour to bypass the pupil (arrows) and so eliminates the iris bombé, hence making the angle less narrow, which is enough to protect against future angle closure.

Accordingly, the pupil is on a more anterior plane than usual, which narrows the angle of the anterior chamber. Gonioscopy is therefore important in diagnosis (see p. 61).

A diabolical feature for closed-angle glaucoma is that *the lens in all eyes (not only CAG eyes) goes on increasing in size throughout life*, the only organ in the body to behave in this way. The resulting gradual shallowing of the anterior chamber is important in a small eyeball for two reasons. First, the angle of the anterior chamber becomes even more narrow. Second, there is increasing resistance to the flow of aqueous humour through the pupil into the anterior chamber ('relative pupil block'): the iris, a very elastic structure, balloons slightly forwards into the anterior chamber (iris bombé), thereby narrowing the angle even more.

This vicious circle progresses and leads to blockage of the trabecular meshwork (p. 53 and Fig. 5.2) by the base of the iris with *either* a sudden attack of acute closed-angle glaucoma (often preceded by subacute attacks in the early evening for a few weeks) *or* a gradual development of chronic closed-angle glaucoma, which is similar to open-angle glaucoma (see below). See Figs 5.13 and 5.14. About 25% of cases of closed-angle glaucoma present as chronic CAG, 75% as acute CAG. The quite common insidious evolution into chronic closed-angle glaucoma probably occurs because the closure of the angle is progressive from above downward (12 o'clock is the narrowest and 6 o'clock is the widest part). See Fig. 5.14. In acute closed-angle glaucoma, the whole angle closes off quite quickly, preventing all escape of aqueous humour quite suddenly with dramatic results. See below and Fig. 5.13.

In recent years evidence for abnormal activity of the sympathetic and parasympathetic nervous system has appeared that may explain why

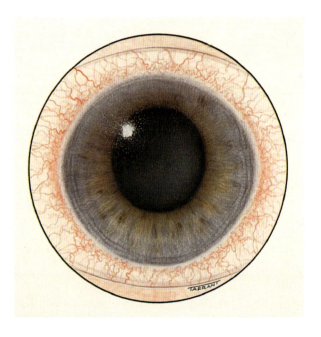

Fig. 5.13. Acute closed-angle glaucoma. The predisposed angle (see Fig. 5.14) has closed completely and suddenly. Quickly, within half an hour or so, the intraocular pressure has risen to 50–60 mmHg (stony-hard and very tender on digital tonometry) with severe pain, often vomiting, poor visual acuity (usually worse than 6/24), a vertically oval, semi-dilated pupil due to shortening of the 12 o'clock sector of the iris, and a 'steamy' cornea (due to multiple droplets of oedema).

acute CAG tends to occur in the early evening (when the anterior chamber is shallower than at other times) and also has a higher seasonal prevalence in the autumn.

Although at first there is merely contact-closure between the periphery of the iris and the trabecular meshwork, this is gradually converted to irreversible fibrous permanent *gonio-synechiae* especially as a result of subacute or acute attacks of closed-angle glaucoma.

Note that in these predisposed eyes, there is a significant risk that mydriatics will produce acute closed-angle glaucoma.

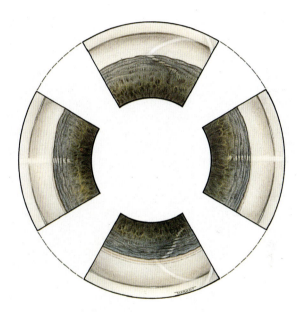

Fig. 5.14. Gonioscopic appearances of the angle of the anterior chamber of an eye about to develop acute closed-angle glaucoma, or insidious chronic closed-angle glaucoma. At 6 o'clock the angle is open and two narrow bands of brownish-red colour can be seen parallel to the base of the iris. The broader one nearer the iris's base is the trabecular meshwork. (The further one is Schwalbe's line.) As the angle is traced upwards it gradually narrows until at 9 and 3 o'clock the base of the iris closes off the trabecular meshwork. That closure involves the upper half of the angle.

ACUTE CLOSED-ANGLE GLAUCOMA

(See Fig. 5.13.) See Table 6.1 for differential diagnosis of the red eye. The evolution of the closure of the angle described above results in acute closed-angle glaucoma in about 75% of cases of angle-closure who often give a history of some subacute attacks in the preceding weeks or month or so. Note that the pressure may be normal between attacks, hence the importance of gonioscopy. These subacute attacks tend to occur in the evening, causing discomfort or even pain in the eye for an hour or two, relieved by going to sleep because the pupil constricts — miosis — in sleep. During the (sub)acute attack, coloured rings around lights ('haloes') are sometimes seen for an hour or so at a time because droplets of fluid appear in the cornea (corneal oedema) in response to a *sudden* rise in intraocular pressure. These droplets refract the various wavelengths constituting white light into separate bundles which are seen as colours (long wavelengths (red) are refracted least; short wavelengths (blue) are refracted most) as in a rainbow. This is not a very reliable symptom because the commonest cause of haloes is early cataract *in which case they are not intermittent.* Open-angle glaucoma is a rare cause of 'haloes', rather surprisingly because (a) the rise of pressure is not usually so acute, even when aggravated by a diurnal (circadian) rhythm, and (b) the rise in pressure is usually not so high as in closed-angle glaucoma.

The acute attack itself is one of the few ophthalmic emergencies, excluding trauma, and is usually easy to diagnose.

Symptoms

- Pain in and around the eye occurs quite suddenly and becomes severe within a few hours.
- The patient may vomit.
- Haloes (coloured rings round lights) may be noticed.

Signs

- Visual acuity is usually reduced to 6/60 or less as a result of *corneal oedema* which makes the cornea semiopaque because of a diffuse multiplicity of tiny droplets of fluid.
- The pupil is semidilated and oval with its long axis vertical (because of shortening of the 12 o'clock sector of the iris); the observer can see this with a good light and close inspection in spite of corneal oedema.
- Digital tonometry (gentle — the eye is very tender) reveals a stony-hard eyeball; see Fig. 5.4. A tonometer reads around 50 mmHg.

Beware of missing less acute or less severe examples in stoical patients who have less acute rises in pressure, quite good or even normal VA, little corneal oedema, and no obvious oval dilatation of the pupil. The irregularly recurrent history should arouse suspicion, supported by a finding of a rather smaller than usual eyeball ('little piggy eye') especially a small diameter cornea and, on closer inspection, a shallow anterior chamber. The 'eclipse test' may help here. Shine a light on to the eye from the temporal side in the same plane as the iris. If the pupil *is* on a more anterior plane than the periphery of the iris, i.e. the anterior chamber is shallow, the nasal side of the iris should be in shadow.

Management

The patient with acute CAG should reach an ophthalmic surgeon as soon as possible, even during the night. Any delay in reducing the very high intraocular pressure increases the risk of permanent damage to the optic disc and permanent gonio-synechiae.

Fellow eye. The other eye is always as important as the affected or presenting eye in all eye diseases. In this case, the fellow eye is anatomically predisposed to the same disease, having come from the same factory. Occasionally acute CAG is bilateral. The fellow eye should be made 'safe', until a prophylactic peripheral iridectomy can be done, by immediately instilling weak pilocarpine eye drops (0.5% or 1%), then, 5 minutes later, a beta-blocker such as timolol 0.5%.

The former is continued every 4 hours and the latter twice daily. Pilocarpine constricts the pupil and so 'pulls' the base of the iris out of the angle of the anterior chamber, while timolol reduces the iris bombé by reducing production of aqueous humour.

'Acute eye'. The objective is to lower the pressure to normal so that an iridectomy or a drainage operation can be done with greater safety than if the operation is done when the pressure is still high.

- Pilocarpine 1%, 2% or, best, 4% eye drops are instilled, then, 5 minutes later, timolol 0.5%. However, these are seldom effective because they fail to penetrate the oedematous cornea.
- Acetazolamide (diamox) 500 mg IV or IM will usually reduce the intraocular pressure to painless levels. This drug can then be continued by mouth.
- Intravenous hypertonic mannitol is usually reserved for 2–3 hours before operation if acetazolamide fails. (It is also used by neurosurgeons to reduce intracranial pressure temporarily).

- Systemic pain-relieving drugs should be given, not excluding an injection of morphine, which has the advantage of encouraging miosis. Vomiting may preclude the oral route.
- Remember that a general anaesthetic may be required within a few hours.

Shortly after the pressure has been made normal, the ophthalmic surgeon must do either (a) a laser or surgical iridectomy or (b) a drainage operation (see Fig. 5.16) depending on the duration of the acute attack, and the surgeon's assessment by gonioscopy of how much of the angle has opened. In the longer term, if these operations fail to control the pressure, a beta-blocker is much preferable to pilocarpine because no aqueous humour now passes through the pupil; the latter drug inevitably causes *all* of the posterior surface of the iris and pupil to press constantly on the lens in the still shallow anterior chamber so that *total* posterior synechiae result (see also p. 88 and Fig. 6.3), probably with a membrane covering the pupil requiring cataract extraction. A repeat drainage operation is less likely to be successful than the first (see Fig. 5.16).

A week or so later the other eye receives its laser iridotomy, or prophylactic peripheral iridectomy surgically, to eliminate the iris bombé. That reduces the narrowness of the angle to a level we know empirically to be safe indefinitely even though the lens still goes on increasing in size. The use of iridectomy presupposes that tonometry has shown the preoperative pressure to be normal and gonioscopy has shown that at least 66 – 75% of the angle is open. Care is required postoperatively: since all the aqueous goes through the iridectomy and none through the pupil, the traumatic postoperative iridocyclitis strongly tends to produce posterior synechiae: preoperative and postoperative topical steroids, and postoperatively a mild mydriatic (e.g. tropicamide 0.5%), usually prevent that. If conservative prophylactic peripheral iridectomy unexpectedly fails to control pressure completely, timolol is much preferable to pilocarpine because the latter drug condemns that eye (i.e. one with an iridectomy through which travels all aqueous humour, bypassing the pupil) to total posterior synechiae, probably with a pupillary membrane necessitating cataract extraction.

Open-angle (Chronic Simple) Glaucoma

Cause
The raised pressure in OAG is the result of an inherited defect in the function of the endothelial cells of the trabecular meshwork: more

precise pathophysiology is unknown. See Figs 5.1 and 5.2. Around 5% of the first-degree relatives over 50 years of age of OAG patients will have OAG also (compare 1% of the general population, although the prevalence rises to as much as 5–8% over 80 years of age). Note the similarity to the heredity of CAG.

Clinical Features
The presenting symptom is usually a report from the optometrist who has been prescribing spectacles for a presbyope and has found a pressure of 23–24 mmHg or more on tonometry. The triad typical of OAG is

1. raised intraocular pressure (≥ 23–24 mmHg);
2. pathological cupping of the optic disc;
3. typical field loss.

Such a patient should be referred urgently to an eye specialist. A family history increases the level of suspicion. However, a raised pressure probably precedes field loss and pathological cupping by several years; all such so-called ocular hypertensives do not necessarily develop OAG, but the authors are cautious enough to prefer to treat many of them. Conversely, and astonishingly, a small proportion of cases have pathological cupping and typical field loss but normal pressure — 'low-tension' or 'normal pressure' glaucoma; various rather unsatisfactory theories have been suggested to explain this, but it is usually treated as for OAG.

When the intraocular pressure rises above 24 mmHg, progressive pathological cupping and field loss are likely to supervene. All these are often symptomless until late in the disease when field loss is severe: early diagnosis depends on the vigilance of optometrists. The field loss is peripheral, so that the patient retains good visual acuity until the late stages of the disease and often fails to notice quite severe field loss, especially if one eye is more affected than the other. The field loss is typical — an arcuate scotoma arching upwards and nasally above fixation from the blind spot, then a superonasal peripheral defect. See Fig. 5.15.

This upper half field loss progresses quite far before the lower half of the field begins to suffer in a similar way. These field changes correlate with disc changes: a physiological cup (cup-disc or C/D ratio of 0.5 or less) enlarges, especially inferiorly, until, at a C/D ratio of 0.75 — the criterion for a 'pathological cup' — the probability of OAG is 65%. Note the more doubtful ratio between 0.5 and 0.75. See Fig. 5.3. The vertical C/D ratio is a more appropriate property than the horizontal one. A difference of 0.2 in the C/D ratio between the right and left eyes is a strong indication of glaucoma, even when both cups are 'physiological'.

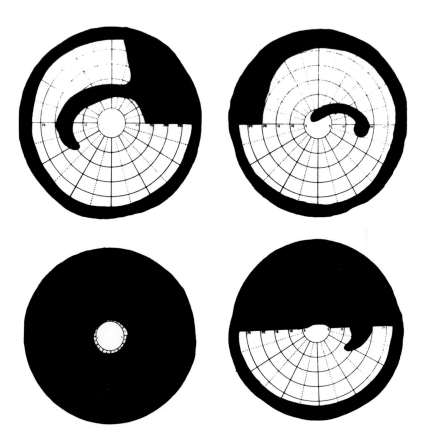

Fig. 5.15. Typical field changes in open-angle (chronic simple) glaucoma. Top right is an early stage in a patient's right eye with an 'arcuate scotoma' arching over towards fixation (the centre point of all the circles) from the blind spot. Note the early 'nasal step' in the periphery of the nasal side of the field. Top left is a more advanced stage in the same patient's left eye: the arcuate scotoma has joined up with a much larger nasal step.

Lower right shows complete loss of the upper half of the right field and the start of an inferior arcuate scotoma from the blind spot. Lower left shows a very advanced stage of glaucoma in the same patient's left eye with only a little more than 5° of the central field remaining: 'tube field' or 'tunnel vision'.

Typical field loss and pathological cupping are enough to make the diagnosis of glaucoma. Gonioscopy will exclude CAG, which is very important because some cases that seem to have OAG (?10%) in fact turn out to have chronic CAG: see p. 67 Slit-lamp examination will exclude iridocyclitis, which is a cause of 'secondary' glaucoma. If the ocular tension on one occasion is not abnormally high, that is no evidence against OAG because diurnal variations in pressure may well allow it to be normal at some time during the day. Accordingly, many ophthalmologists perform tonometry every 3–4 hours during the day ('phasing') but few carry that to its logical conclusion and do 24-hour phasing!

Management

In contrast to the urgent operations to both eyes in CAG, it is common practice to treat OAG medically until and unless there is definite evidence of progressive field loss.

- Recording of fields of vision every 4–6 months is important.
- Timolol 0.25% or 0.5% or other ß-blocker eyedrops are usually the first to be prescribed once or twice daily. These reduce the pressure by reducing the amount of aqueous humour secreted; surprisingly that does not cause cataract. Patients should be instructed to apply pressure over the lower lacrimal canaliculi and keep their eyes shut for five minutes after instillation of the drops. That improves intraocular penetration of the drug through the cornea, and reduces the amount of drug reaching the systemic circulation via the lacrimal ducts and nasal mucosa. The first pass avoids the liver (hence its surprising systemic effect) where the drug is maximally broken down in the second and subsequent passes. Patients with cardiac disease, especially those with bradycardia or in danger of decompensation, and patients with obstructive airways disease should be treated with β-blockers very cautiously if at all, even with selective β_2 blockers (or stimulators, surprisingly) in cardiac cases and selective β_1 blockers in the respiratory cases. Selectivity is seldom exclusive and often not permanent.
- Pilocarpine 0.5% or 1% or 2% eye drops are commonly also prescribed, every 4–6 hours. Unlike in CAG, the objective here is to cause contraction of the ciliary muscle (by a direct effect on the muscle cells), which pulls on its attachment at the scleral spur and trabecular meshwork hence opening up the channels of outflow. An unwanted side-effect (compare CAG) is miosis that darkens vision, sometimes unacceptably. An Ocusert (May & Baker), placed behind the lower eyelid, consists of a membrane of ethylene–vinyl acetate co-polymer, with a matrix of alginic acid which constitutes a reservoir of pilocarpine; the drug remains active continuously for about a week.
- Adrenaline 1% or 2% sometimes with guanethidine, or the pro-

drug dipivefrine HC1 (Propine 0.1%) may be given twice daily, even with a β-blocker! It probably reduces aqueous secretion *and* increases outflow.

- Ophthalmologists are rather reluctant to prescribe acetazolamide, a carbonic anhydrase inhibitor, by mouth long-term because of the effect on electrolytes and the tendency to cause renal calculi. It reduces production of aqueous humour and is additive to the effect of β-blockers. A topical preparation may be available soon.

- If intraocular pressure and field loss are not controlled by maximum tolerable medical treatment, laser trabeculoplasty or drainage

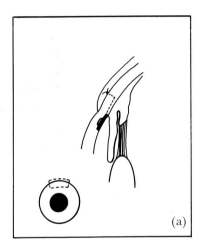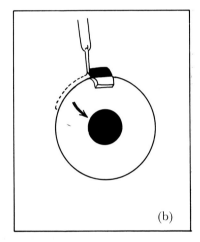

(a)   (b)

Fig. 5.16. (a) Trabeculectomy is currently the standard drainage operation for open-angle (chronic simple) and chronic closed-angle glaucoma. After the usual conjunctival flap has been reflected forwards, a trapdoor of sclera is raised from behind forwards along the dotted line, hinged with the attached base anteriorly (see b); the incision enters the canal of Schlemm (Fig. 5.1) along approximately 5 mm of its length. The trabecular meshwork and some tissue anterior and posterior to it, as shown by the black rectangle, are excised. The scleral trapdoor, then the conjunctival flap, are sutured into place. Aqueous humour probably trickles out round the scleral trapdoor to reach the subconjunctival tissues. (b) Trabeculotomy is done in some centres, e.g. in some cases of congenital glaucoma and in some aphakic eyes with glaucoma. As in trabeculectomy, a scleral flap is raised under a conjunctival flap and the canal of Schlemm is entered along 4 mm or so of its extent. A curved probe (dotted line) attached to a handle is introduced along the canal to one side. The handle is then rotated so that the probe moves in the direction of the arrow into the anterior chamber, thereby breaking down the trabecular meshwork over about one quarter of its extent. The same manoeuvre is done on the other side of the trapdoor to add almost another quarter.

operation (Fig. 5.16) are usually done. (A significant proportion of surgeons, however, favour earlier active intervention.) In laser trabeculoplasty, a fine beam from an argon laser is applied to the trabecular meshwork through a special gonioscope; blanching is produced in continuous spots around part or the whole of the linear extent of the meshwork. Trabeculectomy (a surgical drainage operation) is described in Fig. 5.16. Improvement of the outflow of aqueous humour is the objective of both procedures.

Glaucoma Complicating Other Pathological Processes: Secondary Glaucoma

Iridocyclitis is the usual culprit especially in eyes already predisposed to CAG or OAG because inflammatory exudate from the iris and ciliary body blocks the trabecular meshwork. The main aim of treatment is to reduce the inflammation, usually with topical steroids. Mydriasis with atropine is usually required — unfortunately, since it tends to raise intraocular pressure (compare pilocarpine); adrenaline is often added, which helps mydriasis and reduces IOP. Pilocarpine and other miotics must be avoided, so that acetazolamide by mouth for a few days or weeks may be necessary.

Another mechanism may produce glaucoma in iridocyclitis. As a result of iridocyclitis, the pupil constricts (the ciliary muscle also contracts) and the iris becomes sticky (see also p. 88). There is great danger that the pupil will become bound down irreversibly to the underlying lens: when that process is complete, aqueous cannot reach the anterior chamber and so the iris balloons forwards (iris bombé) much more markedly than in CAG, and its periphery closes the trabecular meshwork, hence producing severe glaucoma that requires urgent iridectomy or drainage operation. The earlier that treatment of the iridocyclitis is started, the less likely is that disastrous outcome.

Steroid glaucoma is a serious risk after 4–6 weeks of topical treatment, at least in those with an hereditary predisposition to OAG. Long-term steroids should only be prescribed under careful ophthalmological supervision. (Actually the same applies to short-term topical steroids because unsuspected dendritic ulcers may well be the cause of a red eye, the usual reason for their being prescribed. Mixtures of antibiotics and steroids are better left to the responsibility of the ophthalmologist, too.) For some unknown reason, steroids reduce the facility of outflow of aqueous humour through the trabecular meshwork.

Concussion of the eyeball may in the longer term be a (forgotten) cause of glaucoma. That cause should be suspected if a glaucoma is unilateral, provided CAG is excluded.

Neovascular glaucoma is a common end-result of central retinal vein occlusion (which is itself an occasional complication of open-angle or closed-angle glaucoma), unless ischaemic retina is converted to dead retina by panretinal photocoagulation. See also p. 97. From ischaemic retina, a neovasculogenic polypeptide diffuses to produce local new vessels in the retina and vitreous (and occasionally vitreous haemorrhage) — as in diabetic retinopathy. Even more disastrously, the substance is carried forward with aqueous humour to stimulate new vessels in the iris and angle of the anterior chamber, which obstruct outflow of aqueous humour to produce a 'blind painful eye' that the patient may ask to have removed. Although standard drainage operations cannot relieve the condition, one end of a fine silicone tube can be inserted surgically into the anterior chamber, under a conjunctival flap, to lead the aqueous outside the eyeball, thereby reducing pressure and eliminating pain (Molteno implant, or a variant).

'Lens-induced glaucoma' is unusual. A mature cataract (see p. 106) exists when lens opacification is complete: the pupil is densely white. By itself, that does not produce glaucoma. 'Hypermaturity' is applied when maturity, usually of long standing, has progressed to (a) swelling ('intumescence') of the lens, which causes a very shallow anterior chamber and blockage of the outflow of aqueous humour by the base of the iris as in acute CAG above (p. 70), or (b) rupture of the thinned lens capsule through which lens matter extrudes to silt up the trabecular meshwork (often with an allergic reaction to lens protein in the angle). Many hypermature lenses merely shrink (and may liquefy) and eventually may dislocate following minor trauma. Even a normal lens may be dislocated following a sudden severe concussion injury to the eyeball. If the dislocated lens moves anteriorly it may have the same effect as an intumescent lens: that is a possible occurrence in Marfan syndrome.

Malignant melanoma of ciliary body, or the base of the iris, may very rarely cause glaucoma by infiltrating the trabecular meshwork throughout most of its extent.

Screening

As previously emphasized, early diagnosis is important in preventing visual loss from glaucoma. Optometrists, seeing presbyopes regularly, provide a very valuable screening service for the most important age group. That is one reason why few ophthalmologists advocate general population screening. A good case can be made out for screening all first-degree relatives over the age of, say, 60 years of patients with OAG and CAG. The history taken by the optometrist or general practitioner should include a question on family history of eye disease. False positives, false negatives and administrative costs make the opportunity costs of this and many other screening services rather high. 'Opportunity cost' is a term used by economists and indicates that when resources are devoted to a certain purpose other possible objectives have to be sacrificed, given that resources are always scarce.

Chapter 6

THE RED EYE

The red eye is a common problem in general practice and accident and emergency departments. Most cases are easy to diagnose and treat, but a few are serious and require urgent referral to a specialist. See Table 6.1. This chapter is planned particularly to differentiate these two groups. For the non-specialist, a high degree of confidence in the diagnosis is possible in the vast majority of cases without a slit-lamp microscope. Its use by the specialist allows even greater precision: the student should take the opportunity in the out-patient department to enjoy the beautiful view of the anterior segment of the eye as seen through the instrument.

A few key points will be emphasized before more systematic consideration.

- History is important, as always — injury, contact lenses?
- A red eye *with reduced visual acuity* usually warrants emergency referral to an eye specialist.
- Visual acuity (VA) is moderately or greatly reduced in acute closed-angle glaucoma (CAG), corneal ulcer and keratitis; moderately reduced in early iridocyclitis; but in conjunctivitis is normal.
- In corneal ulcer, keratitis and acute CAG, close inspection and good illumination will usually reveal a hazy cornea.
- Conjunctivitis causes diffuse superficial hyperaemia overlying the white of the eye: the vessels are mobile when the examiner uses the edge of the lower lid to disturb then. VA is normal.
- Mucopurulent conjunctivitis is bilateral. VA is normal.
- Even in early mild unilateral iridocyclitis the pupil is small compared with the normal side.
- Circumcorneal bluish hyperaemia with immobile vessels (see conjunctivitis above) is typical of iridocyclitis and corneal ulceration.
- Scleritis, which is rare, produces a deep patch of redness: vessels are immobile when the examiner uses the edge of the lower lid to try to disturb them.

Conjunctivitis

Acute Bacterial Conjunctivitis

The patient tells you the diagnosis when he says that his eyelids have been stuck together with muco-pus for the last few mornings and his 'gritty' eyes are producing a watery and pussy discharge in the daytime. There may be a gap of a few hours between the onset in the right and left eyes but this disease is markedly bilateral. The visual acuity is normal. Crusting is usually obvious on the lid margins and eyelashes. Both conjunctivae are diffusely red. The corneae are clear and bright.

The pneumococcus or staphylococcus is probably the commonest pathogen but a swab should be taken for culture before treatment is started. Broad-spectrum antibiotic eye drops (guttae in UK: collyria in USA) should be prescribed immediately and intensively, with, at night, the same drug in an eye ointment (oculentum, *not* unguentum which is a skin ointment). For the first five minutes, the patient should lie flat on a couch, and a relative or friend is shown how to 'dribble' the drops underneath the upper lid to reach the upper conjunctival fornix and into the lower fornix once every minute, avoiding contamination of the tip of the dropper. For the next hour, that treatment is repeated every five minutes. Hourly instillations (into the lower fornix will suffice now) are done for the next 4-5 hours, then drops should be continued every 3 hours for several days. The oculentum generously instilled into the lower fornix at night not only avoids the quick disappearance of the transient therapeutic concentration obtained from eye drops, but prevents the unpleasant crusting of the eyelids in the mornings.

Regarding choice of antibiotic, remember that chloramphenicol (like other drugs, of course) is absorbed into the general circulation and that blood dyscrasias, some fatal, have been reported occasionally, at least from prolonged use: the connection is probably under-diagnosed and under-reported. Several other broad-spectrum antibiotic eye drops and oculenta are available.

The patient and all attendants must apply high standards of hygiene, including a no-touch technique as far as practicable, especially in institutions, throughout the period of treatment. Tubes of ointment and the unused contents of drop bottles should be discarded at the end of treatment to avoid the risk of use of contaminated material on any future occasion.

Acute (muco-)purulent conjunctivitis, bilateral of course, in the newborn ('ophthalmia neonatorum') may be due to *Chlamydia trachomatis* (see p. 183) or the gonococcus *or both*: a female child may also have vulvo-vaginitis. Systemic as well as topical treatment should be used

Table 6.1 Differential diagnosis of the red eye.

Symptoms	Acute closed-angle glaucoma (Fig. 5.13)	Acute iridocyclitis (Fig. 6.3)	Conjunctivitis			Keratitis and corneal ulcers (Figs 6.1 and 6.2)
			Acute bacterial	Acute adenovirus	(Acute) Chlamydial (Figs 15.3 and 15.4)	
Previous history	Episodes of blurring, pain or haloes for an hour or two in some early evenings for a few weeks	Any previous attack protracted for weeks	Possible	Sometimes	Frequent recurrences: *often chronic*	Previous attacks frequent in viral types Foreign body or other injury. Contact lenses
Pain	Severe, radiating to forehead, with vomiting often	Moderate, localized to eye. Dull	Gritty, especially on blinking	Gritty, especially on blinking	Variable discomfort, gritty	Moderate to severe. Sharp on blinking
Photophobia	Slight	Moderate	Slight	Slight/moderate	Variable	*Marked*
Secretion or discharge	Watery	Watery	*(Muco-) purulent: heavy.* Neutrophils	Watery. Monocytes	Watery ± pus Neutrophils *Inclusion bodies*	Watery + + Monocytes in herpes simplex
Visual acuity	*Bad*, usually	Poor or slightly reduced	*Normal*	*Normal*	Normal at first. If chronic, often eventual blindness	*Poor to bad, usually*
Onset	2 – 3 hours	Gradual (1 – 2 days)	Within 1 – 2 days	Several days	Several days	Gradual (1 – 2 days)
Systemic symptoms	Often prostration and vomiting because of pain	Usually none	None	None	None	None
Bilateral?	Unilateral usually	Unilateral usually	*Invariably bilateral*	Unilateral or bilateral	Bilateral (at first may be unilateral)	Unilateral usually
Age	Usually 50 +	Usually 15 – 25	Any, but usually in children	Any, but usually up to 25	Any	Any

	Acute closed-angle glaucoma (Fig 5.13)	Acute iridocyclitis (Fig 6.3)	Conjunctivitis — Acute bacterial	Conjunctivitis — Acute adenovirus	(Acute) Chlamydial (Figs 15.3 and 15.4)	Keratitis and corneal ulcers (Figs 6.1 and 6.2)
Signs						
Hyperaemia	Circumcorneal purple + diffuse conjunctival	Circumcorneal purple + diffuse conjunctival	Conjunctival, severe and diffuse. Brick red	Conjunctival, mild. Often restricted to a sector next to limbus	Diffuse conjunctival	Circumcorneal purple
Cornea	Epithelial oedema (fogged view of iris)	(Keratic) precipitates	Clear and sparkling	Looks clear but fluorescein stains 'superficial punctate' spots, seen with slit-lamp microscope	Clear. Late: *pannus and/or diffuse fibrosis, also of conjunctiva*	*Grey area and/or stains* with fluorescein. *Dendritic* pattern in herpes simplex
Anterior chamber	*Shallow* (N.B. see fellow eye)	*Exudate (flare; cells)* Often deep. Sometimes hypopyon	Normal	Normal	Normal	As in iridocyclitis. Hypopyon sometimes
Iris	Oedematous and hyperaemic	Often hyperaemic and 'muddy'	Normal	Normal	Normal	Usually hyperaemic
Pupil	*Dilated, oval*	Contracted	Normal	Normal	Normal	Usually concentrated
Pupil light reflex	Absent or reduced	Reduced or absent	Normal	Normal	Normal	Reduced or absent if visible
Tension	Very high	High, normal or low	Normal	Normal	Normal	Usually normal to low
Tenderness	Marked	Moderate to marked	Slight	Slight	Slight	Marked
Other points	Parent or sibling may have had emergency eye operation	Ankylosing spondylitis in males sometimes	Epidemic in school or family?	Pre-auricular lymph node swollen and tender. Epidemic at school or work?	In newborn, mother ± father have GU infection. See trachoma p. 183	History of injury often

and an immediate search of the mother's *and* father's genito-urinary tracts made to find the source(s). Treatment for all three requires collaboration with a specialist in genito-urinary medicine, but see pp. 183–189 which deal with trachoma and its initiating 'inclusion conjunctivitis'.

Adenovirus Conjunctivitis

A more accurate term is kerato-conjunctivitis since the cornea usually shows on slit-lamp microscopy a scattering of small spots of epithelial involvement that stain with fluorescein. Surprisingly, it is predominantly or entirely unilateral: the eye is (slightly) watery and the conjunctiva is diffusely or sectorally hyperaemic. A pre-auricular lymph node may be enlarged and tender. Visual acuity is usually unaffected. An antibiotic oculentum is prescribed 2–3 times daily to lubricate away some of the 'grittiness', although it has no effect on the organism. To prevent spread, hygiene is again important for the patient, but even more so for the nurses and doctors in (ophthalmic) A & E departments and clinics.

Allergic Conjunctivitis

Allergic conjunctivitis associated with hay fever, asthma or exposure to a known allergen is easy to diagnose: diffuse or patchy bilateral redness and watering are typical. Antihistamine eye drops work well. A particular form, vernal or spring catarrh, is commoner in tropical countries and can be chronic and disabling with a troublesome itch in spite of treatment with cromoglycate (which may fail) or steroids (subject to monitoring of intra-ocular pressure). A typical feature is lumpy cobblestones of the conjunctiva under the upper lid, which can often be seen from below without everting the upper lid (to be avoided if possible in children). In severe cases, the cornea may be involved.

Occasionally, *chemosis* (oedematous conjunctiva that may be marked enough to protrude forwards between the eyelids) will alarm the patient unduly: an oculentum and taping down of the upper eyelid to support the conjunctiva and cover the cornea will usually avoid complications until resolution occurs.

Allergy to the active constituent or the vehicle in eye drops or oculenta is quite often the explanation for (bilateral) red, scaly lids or, in severe cases, markedly oedematous eyelids. (A similar complication in the skin elsewhere can occur with unguenta, i.e. ointments for external application.) Topical penicillin is never used in ophthalmology because it carries a high risk.

Acute Haemorrhagic Conjunctivitis

Acute haemorrhagic conjunctivitis has occurred in outbreaks mainly in Africa and the Far East. In a high proportion of cases, petechial or blotchy conjunctival haemorrhages are added to the usual bilateral watering, hyperaemia and mucopurulent discharge. Malaise is common, and a poliomyelitis-like systemic disease affects some cases. A picornavirus is the probable cause.

Subconjunctival Haemorrhage

Subconjunctival haemorrhage is not rare and occurs in the elderly. The patient may be alarmed to see in the mirror a striking large bluish-red area of 'spontaneous' haemorrhage that has obscured much of the sclera ('white of the eye'). There is seldom any history of injury or disease predisposing to haemorrhage, and there are usually no symptoms whatsoever (occasionally negligible discomfort). The patient can almost invariably be reassured that it is of no serious significance, even if recurrent, and will disappear in a week or so, as will any bruise.

Herpetic Keratitis (Dendritic Ulcer): Herpes Simplex Virus (Fig. 6.1)

A unilateral red watering eye, especially in a child, should be assumed to have a corneal ulcer due to the virus of herpes simplex until definitely proved otherwise, even if visual acuity is normal. Proof depends on instilling fluorescein eye drops, the excess being washed out with sterile saline (N.B. use a single-dose formulation to avoid cross-infection); close inspection, preferably with magnification, and a bright light, preferably blue, will reveal one or more thin linear branching (hence 'dendritic') superficial fluorescent ulcers without surrounding infiltrate somewhere on the cornea (see Fig. 6.1). Early treatment with acyclovir 3% eye ointment (*Zovirax*, Wellcome) usually cures. *Steroid eye drops must be avoided in such cases even if the diagnosis of dendritic ulcer is merely possible.*

If topical steroids are used, the pain diminishes but the ulcer(s) multiply and spread (a) widely on the surface of the cornea to produce a sloughy 'geographical ulcer' or (b) deeply into the corneal stroma to produce a 'disciform keratitis'; both are disastrous complications that may well occur without steroids. In *disciform keratitis*, not necessarily but usually immediately preceded by dendritic ulcers, a central area of cornea, 3–7mm in diameter, becomes greyish-white, opaque and thickened with loss of corneal epithelium. The corneal endothelium is also usually involved. Inflammatory toxins diffuse into the aqueous humour and cause iridocyclitis. Pain is constant and severe. The eventual end-result after months of disabling symptoms is a white corneal scar that has a poor prognosis for corneal grafting because of heavy vascularization. Fortunately, it is practically always unilateral. The strong tendency for dendritic ulcers to recur 'spontaneously', or following minor local trauma or reduced general resistance, is explained by the unfortunate ability of the cornea to nurture latent virus and quite probably by chronic infection of the trigeminal ganglion (as in herpes zoster ophthalmicus, for which there is better evidence; see p. 158).

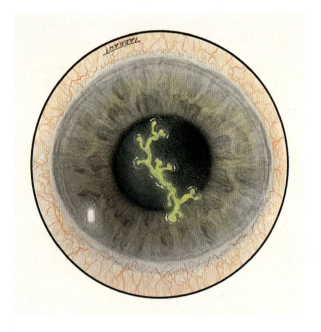

Fig. 6.1. Very large obvious dendritic ulcer stained with fluorescein eye drops, excess washed off with 2 – 3 drops of saline. Originally it was tiny, but was aggravated by steroid eye drops wrongly prescribed for an undiagnosed unilateral 'red sore eye'.

Other corneal ulcers

Other corneal ulcers, e.g. due to infection following a corneal foreign body, or unsterile attempts at its removal, are usually easier to diagnose because a grey-white slough is usually quite obvious on close inspection with a bright light of a painful, watering eye. See Fig. 6.2. Visual acuity is usually reduced. Toxins from the infecting pyogens diffuse through aqueous humour to excite an inflammation in the iris, sometimes severe enough to produce an hypopyon — accumulation of pus cells at the bottom of the anterior chamber (Fig. 6.2). This emergency requires immediate swab and culture to identify pathogens, followed immediately by systemic, topical and subconjunctival antibiotics.

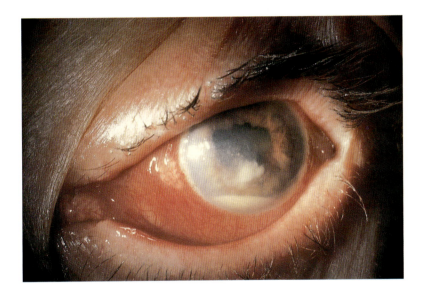

Fig. 6.2. Corneal ulcer following small corneal foreign body although it was removed with sterile precautions. Note the irregularly dilated pupil (following atropine 1% and phenylephrine 10% eye drops) due to posterior synechiae of the pupil to the lens, the result of 'secondary' iritis. Also note hypopyon with fluid level: pus cells from the iris have gravitated downwards.

Agricultural injuries tend to be associated with fungus infections that evolve more slowly without hypopyon but are more difficult to eradicate. A fungus keratitis is an occasional complication of contact lens wear.

Iridocyclitis (Fig. 6.3)

In the perspective of injuries, conjunctivitis, etc., iridocyclitis is a rare cause of the red eye but must not be missed. It is the spot diagnosis in a patient with ankylosing spondylitis and a red eye. Severity of the redness and watering varies widely: often they are quite mild, with only a slight ache. The redness may not be restricted to the circumcorneal region where, however, it tends to be maximal. A good clue is a small

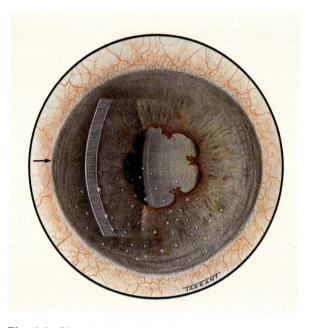

Fig. 6.3. Chronic iridocyclitis, showing about six obvious points where the pupil is stuck to the underlying lens (posterior synechiae): other areas of the pupil have partially dilated in response to atropine 1% and phenylephrine 10% eye drops. Note circumcorneal hyperaemia. The beam of the slit-lamp microscope from the observer's left (arrow) shows white 'keratic precipitates' ('KP') scattered over the *endothelial* surface of the *lower* half of the cornea: these are inflammatory aggregates gravitationally deposited from aqueous humour where they can be seen as bright glistening dots (as in a shaft of light entering a dusty room). The anterior chamber is not optically empty for another reason: the slit beam can be seen traversing it ('flare') because subcellular inflammatory exudate in the aqueous humour scatters some light in the beam. Flare, KP and posterior synechiae are diagnostic of iridocyclitis.

pupil on the affected side, but a definite diagnosis depends on the slit-lamp microscope, which reveals glinting white cells circulating in the aqueous of the anterior chamber: they agglutinate and sediment to produce the diagnostic 'keratic precipitates' (KP) on the back of the lower cornea — sometimes visible to the observer's naked eye. In severe cases, an hypopyon is present (especially in Behçet's disease; see p. 196). The intraocular pressure may be raised but the semidilated oval pupil of closed-angle glaucoma is usually enough to indicate the latter diagnosis. Visual acuity may be normal but more usually is slightly reduced, occasionally greatly. A battery of investigations is often ordered but seldom produces positive results: the occasional case of ankylosing spondylitis can usually be diagnosed on clinical grounds (to avoid unnecessary radiographs especially near the gonads). Sarcoidosis is an occasional cause, especially in low-grade bilateral cases. The condition tends to recur at long intervals.

Disaster can arise from delay in treatment because the sticky inflamed iris is bound down to the underlying lens by posterior synechiae. See Fig. 6.3. Ring synechiae at the pupil can become established quite quickly, completely blocking entry of aqueous humour into the anterior chamber. The iris becomes hugely ballooned forwards (iris bombé), and its base suddenly blocks the trabecular meshwork, hence acute 'secondary' glaucoma. See also p. 77. That in turn requires emergency iridectomy (by laser or surgery) ± drainage operation. Early treatment of iridocyclitis with intensive atropine, phenylephrine and topical steroids is designed to prevent and/or eliminate posterior synechiae by dilating and moving the pupil, and diminishing the inflammatory reaction. Subconjunctival injections of some drugs, especially steroids, may be valuable.

Rosacea

A rare cause of recurrent spells of a few days of redness and watering of either or both eyes in the older patient can be rosacea even if the facial skin is only mildly affected and there is no rhinophyma. A typical pattern of slight superficial peripheral corneal opacification with some thinning and vascularization can eventually be seen with the slit-lamp microscope. Surprisingly, a six-week course of oxytetracycline by mouth, repeated occasionally if necessary, is effective. Topical steroids can be used with some benefit but further thinning with perforation is a risk, as well as glaucoma.

Acute closed-angle glaucoma: see Chapter 5, p. 70 and Fig. 5.13.

Chapter 7

SUDDEN PAINLESS LOSS OF VISION

Loss of vision may be classified according to the rate of onset, either sudden or gradual, with different causative factors predisposing to each individual disease. Acute, painless loss of function in any part of the body usually has a vascular cause, with transient or permanent impairment of the blood supply to the affected tissue. Consistently, the commonest causes of sudden painless loss of vision are usually vascular:

- amaurosis fugax, i.e. transient loss or obscuration of vision for seconds or a few minutes, usually in one eye;
- retinal artery occlusion: central retinal artery or branch retinal artery;
- retinal vein occlusion: central retinal vein or branch retinal vein;
- retinal complications of systemic hypertension;
- giant cell arteritis;
- anterior ischaemic optic neuropathy;
- optic neuritis;
- vitreous haemorrhage;
- papilloedema.

A brief account of the blood supply to the eye will help the understanding of the pathological mechanisms that predispose to sudden painless loss of vision.

Applied Anatomy

The ophthalmic artery arises from the internal carotid artery near the cavernous sinus, and passes into the orbit through the bony optic canal, lying close to the optic nerve. It constitutes the main blood supply to the eye and ocular adnexa. The branches supplying the globe are the following.

- The central retinal artery, supplying the inner layers of the retina. The central retinal artery enters the optic nerve 12–15 mm behind the eyeball, and both 'penetrate' the eyeball at the optic disc or nerve head. At or near the optic disc, the artery divides into four main branches to supply the four quadrants of the retina. *The central retinal artery is an end-artery, i.e. there are normally no effective anastomoses between this vessel and any other.* As the central retinal artery supplies most of the retina, occlusion of this vessel quickly causes acute, severe and permanent retinal damage (Fig. 7.1).

- The short posterior ciliary arteries supplying the optic disc and the choroid. The choroid in turn nourishes the outer retinal layers, including the photoreceptor layer. Note the blood supply to the optic disc because it is important in giant cell arteritis and anterior ischaemic optic neuropathy (below).

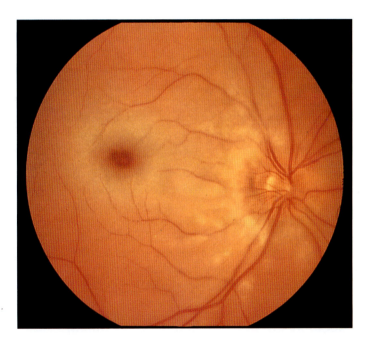

Fig. 7.1. Occlusion of the central retinal artery, usually due to atherosclerosis at the level of the disc. An ischaemic infarct of the retina results from blockage of this end-artery, hence whitish appearance from disc to beyond the macula, and especially around the macula where the retina is thick. At the macula itself the retina is very thin, so that the choroidal blood can be seen easily — 'cherry-red spot'. See Fig. 1.1. The peripheral retina is also thin enough to allow choroidal redness to be seen. The retinal arterioles are thin and obscured in places by some of the patches of retinal oedema or exudates.

Venous drainage of the retina follows a similar pattern to that of the arterial supply, with four main branch retinal veins lying in close apposition to the branch retinal arterioles. These branch veins unite at the optic disc to form the central retinal vein, which leaves the eye close to the central retinal artery through the optic disc and nerve, before eventually draining to the cavernous sinus. The close anatomical proximity of retinal arteries and veins is relevant in the pathogenesis of several ocular conditions.

The pathogenic mechanisms of vascular impairment are the same as in any other part of the body and are, in principle, quite simple. Consider the site of obstruction in relation to the vessel wall.

- *Within the lumen of the blood vessel.* Emboli can cause occlusion, often aggravated by local vasospasm. Also, any increased viscosity of blood constituents, for example in leukaemia and polycythaemia, will increase the risk of stasis.
- *Within the blood vessel wall.* The wall of the blood vessel may be occluded either gradually by atherosclerosis (which can be exacerbated by an overlying thrombus), or acutely by inflammation of the vessel, in arteritis for example.
- *Extrinsic compression of the blood vessel.* This is a relatively common cause of retinal vein occlusion. An adjacent artery may compress the vessel, for example in systemic hypertension and atherosclerosis.

The degree of retinal injury is directly related to the duration of ischaemia in the earliest stages of vascular occlusion. Of course, several hours of ischaemia will cause irreversible damage. Apart from amaurosis fugax, in conditions discussed below, the amount of residual damage can vary dramatically depending on the site of obstruction and for how long the tissue is ischaemic. Some, but not all, conditions are amenable to immediate treatment, so that a quick differential diagnosis is vital to prevent further visual loss — and in some instances blindness.

Aetiology of Sudden Painless Loss of Vision

Amaurosis Fugax

Amaurosis fugax is defined as an episode or, frequently, episodes of transient, uniocular (rarely bilateral) visual loss that is of short duration, usually a few seconds to several minutes; vision recovers fully within 20–30 minutes. The commonest cause is probably platelet–fibrin microemboli that originate from atherosclerotic plaques in the carotid arteries, especially at the origin of the internal carotid artery. Diseased heart valves are a less common source. There is seldom any clinical sign on examination of the retina, as the emboli rapidly disintegrate in the retinal circulation. The diagnosis usually has to be made from the history because carotid bruits or cardiac murmurs may not be found.

Treatment
The underlying cause should be treated after cardiovascular examination. The commonest treatment is anti-platelet agents (e.g. aspirin), but carotid endarterectomy may be indicated in a small proportion of cases.

Central Retinal Artery Occlusion

Occlusion of the central retinal artery quickly causes severe visual loss. See Fig. 7.1.

Pathogenesis
The commonest causes of central retinal artery occlusion are

- thrombosis superimposed on an atherosclerotic plaque;
- emboli (platelet–fibrin, calcific, or cholesterol) originating from the carotid arteries or the heart;
- arteritis, including occasionally giant cell arteritis (but see separate section below).

Signs
- There is profound visual loss (frequently to counting fingers or hand movements) in the affected eye, with unchanged vision in the contralateral eye.
- Pupil reactions demonstate evidence of an afferent pupillary defect, i.e. the pupil in the affected eye will show a diminished or absent reaction to direct light stimulation (the direct response), but light into the contralateral eye will produce a normal response in *both* eyes (the consensual response).
- Ophthalmoloscopy is usually diagnostic. The retina appears pale, almost white, with a characteristic 'cherry-red spot' at the macula; as the retina at the macula is very thin, the macula is transparent to the red colour of underlying choroidal blood. Arteries and veins are attenuated, and there is segmentation within the retinal arteries ('cattle-trucking'). Occasionally, an embolus may be seen within the central retinal artery.

Treatment
Treatment is usually ineffective. Digital massage of the globe and intravenous acetazolamide may be used to lower intraocular pressure, which may improve retinal perfusion. The predisposing cardiovascular cause of the occlusion should be investigated, and giant-cell arteritis excluded. Although the latter is an uncommon cause of central retinal artery occlusion, it may cause rapid-onset *total* blindness, i.e. the other eye may also soon be affected, and therefore must always be considered in the differential diagnosis (see below). An urgent ESR (erythrocyte sedimentation rate) should be performed in all cases of central retinal artery occlusion to exclude giant-cell arteritis. (See separate section below.)

Branch Retinal Artery Occlusion

Occlusion of the temporal retinal arterioles produces more significant effects on vision than occlusion of the nasal branches, as the macula is usually involved. The more peripheral the point of occlusion, the less the effect on visual acuity.

Pathogenesis
Branch retinal arterial occlusion is usually caused by systemic emboli that become lodged in the retinal arterioles. As in central retinal artery occlusion (above), the emboli are of three main types:

- platelet–fibrin emboli, originating usually from the surface of atherosclerotic plaques in the carotid arteries;
- calcific emboli, from diseased cardiac valves;
- cholesterol emboli, arising from atheroma of the carotid arteries.

Symptoms
Symptoms vary from 'amaurosis fugax' (see above) with full visual recovery resulting from small platelet–fibrin emboli that rapidly disintegrate, to severe permanent visual loss following occlusion of temporal retinal arterioles with macular involvement.

Signs

- Pupil responses are not affected: direct and consensual pupil responses are normal.
- Ophthalmoscopy frequently reveals the embolus lodged in the arteriole. There may be significant pallor and oedema of the retina distal to the obstruction in the initial stages.

Treatment

Treatment is similar to that of central retinal artery occlusion, with immediate digital occular massage, which is seldom successful. Assessment of the cardiovascular system is essential to determine the predisposing causes. Antiplatelet agents (e.g. aspirin) may be prescribed, but their long-term benefits have not been established.

Central Retinal Vein Occlusion (See Figs 7.2 and 7.3)

Occlusion of the central retinal vein occurs at the optic disc. Vision is reduced to around 6/60 or less in the affected eye usually over a period of several hours, in marked contrast to central retinal artery occlusion where the visual loss occurs in seconds to minutes.

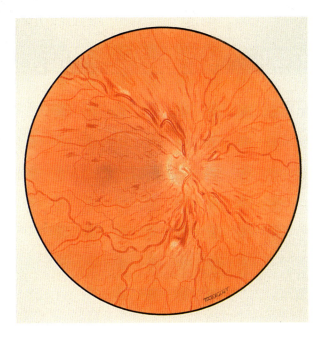

Fig. 7.2. Papilloedema due to central retinal vein occlusion with haemorrhages and exudates scattered widely over the retina: compare Fig. 7.5. Fig. 7.3. shows a more severe occlusion. Visual acuity is usually poor.

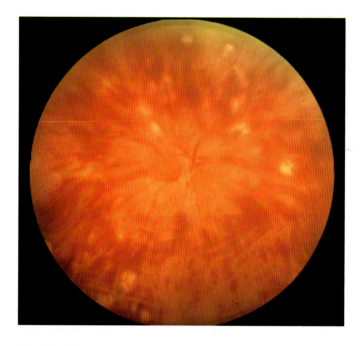

Fig. 7.3. The optic disc in severe central retinal vein occlusion with marked haemorrhages (which also spread widely in the retina, not shown). Visual acuity is very poor in this case. Compare Figs 7.2 and 7.5.

Pathogenesis
Factors are

- external compression of the vein from an atherosclerotic central retinal artery; compression is greater in the presence of arterial hypertension;
- glaucoma;
- hyperviscosity of blood causing venous stasis, e.g. leukaemia, polycythaemia, macroglobulinaemia.

Signs
The retinal appearance on ophthalmoscopy is dramatic and diagnostic: once seen, never forgotten. See Figs 7.2 and 7.3.

- In the acute stage, the retina is obliterated by extensive haemorrhages from disc to periphery, with a particular preponderance of flame-shaped haemorrhages in the nerve fibre layer.

- There is oedema of the optic disc and retina, with gross macular involvement.
- Cottonwool spots are frequently present, indicating retinal ischaemia.

These changes gradually resolve to a variable degree over a period of several months.

Management
There is no effective cure for central retinal vein occlusion. The objective is to search for a predisposing factor and to minimize the risk of severe complications.

Investigation of the predisposing cause. A cardiovascular examination is required, with particular emphasis on the identification of potentially treatable predisposing conditions, e.g. hypertension and diabetes mellitus. Ocular tension must be assessed and gonioscopy performed to exclude glaucoma; *the other eye must also be carefully examined with the same objective.* Leukaemia or other blood dyscrasias may occasionally be responsible; even more rarely a hyperviscosity syndrome may be found.

Complications of central retinal vein occlusion. Ischaemic (but not atrophic) retina is the source of a polypeptide that diffuses throughout the eyeball and stimulates new vessel formation. In about 50% of cases new blood vessels (neovascularization) will develop in the optic disc and retina, and also in the iris (rubeosis iridis) and in the angle of the anterior chamber; this last produces a severe, painful ('neovascular' or 'secondary') glaucoma that necessitates enucleation in a proportion of cases. See also p. 78. The development of neovascularization usually occurs within three months of the venous occlusion in around 50% of patients. Early evidence of ischaemia of the retina is obtained by fundus fluorescein angiography. Patients with central retinal vein occlusion should be closely monitored for 3–6 months following the episode to identify the development of these early new blood vessels, which will usually regress in response to panretinal laser photocoagulation of the retina (see Chapter 10). If new blood vessels in the retina remain untreated, they may rupture, causing haemorrhage into the vitreous with possible fibrosis and subsequent retinal detachment. (*Although central and branch retinal vein occlusion is a significant cause of vitreous haemorrhage, remember that rupture of a blood vessel crossing a retinal hole that is about to cause a retinal detachment is equally common and must be excluded* — see p. 115). The most important principle in the management of central retinal vein occlusion is therefore identification and preventive treatment of predisposing causes, and close monitoring in the immediate post-occlusive period with intervention when required.

Branch Retinal Vein Occlusion (See Fig. 7.4)

This is more common than occlusion of the central retinal vein. Occlusion of a temporal branch often affects the macular area with significant loss of central and peripheral vision. When a nasal vein is affected, there is no central and less peripheral field loss. The site of obstruction is important: the more proximal the lesion, the greater the visual loss. Symptoms may therefore vary from severe visual impairment following proximal occlusion of a temporal retinal vein, to minimal symptoms (or none) in peripheral obstruction of a nasal vessel.

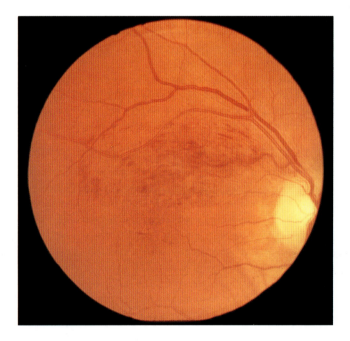

Fig. 7.4. Occlusion of a tributary venule supero-temporal to the right optic disc at a point where an arteriole crosses it. Haemorrhages due to back-pressure affect the venule's territory, which includes the macular area, hence the presenting symptom of sudden painless loss of vision.

Pathogenesis
The causes are similar to those of central retinal vein occlusion, with particular emphasis on external compression of the vein from the accompanying artery at 'crossing-points'. See Fig. 7.4.

Signs

Ophthalmoscopy reveals flame-shaped haemorrhages in one quadrant of the retina (compare central retinal vein occlusion with widespread haemorrhages all over the retina; see Figs 7.2 and 7.3).

Treatment

Predisposing causes and potential complications should be considered as for central retinal vein occlusion. However, neovascularization is uncommon following branch vein occlusion, but if it occurs, photocoagulation is applied to the affected quadrant of the retina.

Retinal Complications of Systemic Hypertension

Although systemic hypertension is discussed in this chapter on sudden painless loss of vision, by itself it seldom produces visual symptoms. However, it predisposes to retinal vascular complications that often do cause sudden loss of vision, especially when the macular area is involved. These are mentioned briefly below. Peripheral retinal vascular lesions may produce small defects in the peripheral field not noticed by the patient.

Applied Anatomy

Raised blood pressure is associated with predictable effects on the retina that are amenable to logical interpretation. The principal factors determining the retinal appearance are firstly the age of the patient, then the level of hypertension, the rate at which the hypertension has developed, and the pre-existing condition of the blood vessels. The arteriolar wall in youth is muscular, with a significant elastic component. As age increases, arteriosclerosis develops, and the normal elements of the vascular wall are gradually replaced by inelastic connective tissue, a process that is accelerated by systemic hypertension. When muscular and elastic tissue are replaced — an irreversible process — the normal constrictive responses of blood vessels to elevation of blood pressure are obviously no longer possible, and the vessels behave like semi-rigid pipes. If blood pressure remains elevated, focal degenerative changes in the vessel walls occur and the vessel leaks, which is disastrous for the retina.

Signs

- In young patients, for example in accelerated (malignant) hypertension, in some renal diseases or in toxaemia of pregnancy, the earliest signs of severe hypertension are usually generalized but there is focal arteriolar constriction causing variations in vessel calibre. (In the elderly, these signs are seldom present because the hypertension has usually developed over a period of years, along with significant underlying arteriosclerosis; accordingly there is insufficient residual muscle and elastin in the vessel wall to allow significant vasoconstriction.)

- Cottonwool spots result from occlusion of arterioles that causes retinal ischaemia.
- Retinal oedema, haemorrhages (typically flame-shaped because in the nerve fibre layer) and hard exudates are due to leakage from damaged vessels.

Changes vary from minimal to severe, depending on the degree, duration, and rate of elevation of blood pressure in the individual patient.

Potential Complications of Systemic Hypertension

- *Branch retinal vein occlusion.* See p. 98. Retinal arterioles and veins share the adventitial sheath at crossing points, so that arterial hypertension causes external compression on the adjacent vein, thereby increasing the risk of vein occlusion. See Fig. 7.4.
- *Central retinal vein occlusion.* See p. 95. This probably occurs by a similar process of external compression on the vein from the adjacent artery. Figs 7.2 and 7.3.
- *Macular exudates.* Leakage of vascular contents from damaged retinal arterioles causes hard exudates to accumulate in the retina. Unfortunately, the macula — and particularly its central area, the fovea — is the most susceptible area in the retina to exudation, and hard exudates within the fovea cause a precipitous decrease in central vision that is usually permanent.
- *Central retinal artery occlusion.* See p. 93; Fig. 7.1.
- *IVth, VIth and (usually partial) IIIrd nerve palsies.* Systemic hypertension, in association with atherosclerosis, is thought to be a common cause of acute nerve palsies, which usually resolve spontaneously within a few weeks.
- *Bilateral optic disc oedema.* Severe acute-onset systemic hypertension may, in a young person, progress to cause bilateral optic disc oedema (papilloedema). See Fig. 7.5. If the hypertension remains untreated, optic atrophy is inevitable.

Treatment

Treatment is obviously directed at the underlying cause. All except the earliest ocular changes of hypertension are irreversible.

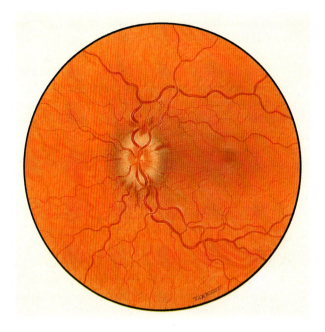

Fig. 7.5. Papilloedema due to raised intracranial pressure (compare Figs 7.2 and 7.3). The optic disc is raised and 'juicy': note the characteristic blurred disc margins and the small haemorrhage (supero-temporally). The oedema is restricted to the disc itself, including its margins, and the remainder of the retina is normal. Visual acuity is normal.

Giant Cell Arteritis

Giant cell arteritis is an (ocular) emergency, and must be excluded in every case of sudden painless loss of vision. The condition was previously known as temporal arteritis, but this term is misleading as giant cell arteritis is an inflammatory disease of large- and medium-diameter arteries which is not restricted to the temporal arteries; generalized arteritis is frequently present at diagnosis. It is a disease of ageing, very seldom occurring in patients of less than 60 years.

Symptoms
The patient frequently presents with acute-onset unilateral profound loss of vision, although systemic constitutional symptoms (malaise, fever, weight loss) may have been present for some weeks or months

prior to the loss of vision. Characteristic symptoms include severe headache associated with tenderness of parts of the temporal arteries and jaw claudication.

Pathogenesis
Giant cell arteritis is a generalized disease, with frequent involvement of coronary, intracranial and renal arteries. In the eye, although it may affect the ophthalmic and central retinal arteries, *the predominant effect is on the posterior ciliary vessels, which causes ischaemic infarction of the optic disc.* The inflammatory process extends through all layers of the artery with lymphocytes, epithelioid cells and mutinucleated giant cells.

Signs
There is an afferent pupillary defect (i.e. impairment or absence of the direct light response in the affected eye, with normal consensual response to light stimulation in the other eye).

The appearance of the optic disc on ophthalmoscopy varies depending on which arteries are particularly affected in the individual patient. The commonest appearance in the acute stage is of a pale, ischaemic, oedematous optic disc with multiple, small splinter haemorrhages, resulting from occlusion of the short posterior ciliary arteries that supply the optic nerve head. Over a period of several weeks the oedema gradually subsides, leaving the characteristic pallor of optic atrophy.

Significant elevation of the erythrocyte sedimentation rate (ESR), often over 70 mm in one hour, is almost diagnostic in giant cell arteritis given the other symptoms. An urgent ESR should be done in all suspected cases of central retinal artery occlusion. A small proportion of cases of giant cell arteritis have a normal ESR for their age. Although biopsy of the temporal artery is often done to confirm the diagnosis, there is a false negative rate of about 10%. The reason is that a normal segment of artery may be obtained since the disease may affect only patches of the arteries — 'skip' lesions. The decision to treat or not must be made very urgently, before the pathological report can be available, because of the high risk to the fellow eye.

Treatment
- *The extreme urgency of this situation cannot be overemphasized because the other eye may be affected at any moment.*
- Systemic steroids in sufficient dosage will prevent involvement of the other eye.
- Intravenous, then oral, systemic steroids are given in high dosage until the oral drug has attained therapeutically effective levels.

- The dosage of steroids is gradually decreased over a period of many weeks or several months, with careful monitoring of the ESR and of systemic side-effects, especially peptic ulceration, hypertension, diabetes, osteoporosis and any infections.
- The maintenance dose may be required for around 1–3 years: N.B. side-effects as above.
- The cardivascular system should be assessed to identify involvement of other arteries for which preventive treatment may be possible.

Anterior Ischaemic Optic Neuropathy (AION)

This is a condition of middle-aged and elderly patients in which ischaemia of the optic nerve head produces sudden painless loss of vision.

Pathogenesis
Anterior ischaemic optic neuropathy is caused by obstruction of the short posterior ciliary arteries at the optic disc, usually because of atherosclerosis (not an arteritic process).

Signs
The signs are dependent on the degree and site of ischaemia. When the ischaemia is predominantly retrobulbar, there may be no abnormality in disc appearance ophthalmoscopically; more commonly, the disc itself is affected and shows pallor with some oedema. Frequently, infarction of the optic nerve head is segmental, producing correspondingly segmental loss of the visual field, e.g. an altitudinal field defect (loss of upper or lower half). The residual disc appearance may demonstrate segmental atrophy consistent with the field defect. Fundus fluorescein angiography demonstrates the segmental decrease in disc perfusion.

Treatment
Giant cell arteritis must always be considered (ESR advisable) before the diagnosis of ischaemic optic neuropathy is made. There is no effective treatment for anterior ischaemic optic atrophy, but a search is made for predisposing causes to prevent further visual loss, e.g. systemic atherosclerosis, hypertension, diabetes mellitus and even syphilis.

Optic Neuritis

Optic neuritis is an important cause of sudden painless visual loss (see p. 124).

Vitreous Haemorrhage

Acute haemorrhage into the vitreous is an uncommon cause of sudden painless loss of vision in non-diabetic subjects. It may result from:

- diabetes mellitus (described in Chapter 10);
- retinal tear or detachment (described on p. 115); this is an important cause and should be considered in all cases to ensure early treatment;
- central or branch retinal vein occlusion (see pp. 95–96 and 98–99);
- blood dyscrasias (rare);
- sickle-cell disease (see below);
- Eales's disease (see below);
- subarachnoid haemorrhage;
- perforating injury;
- concussion of the eye;
- head injury (concussion ± fractured skull). As a result of the sudden rise in intracranial pressure, transmitted down the extension of the subararchnoid space around the optic nerves, sudden back-pressure on the central retinal veins behind the optic discs may cause unilateral or bilateral localised *pre-retinal* haemorrhages (with a horizontal fluid level when the recovered patient is erect): one or both may explode into the vitreous body itself.

SICKLE-CELL DISEASE

Some abnormal haemoglobins alter the normal oval form of the erythrocyte to a crescentic or 'sickle' shape in hypoxia and acidosis. The deformed red blood cells are more rigid than their oval counterparts, and they may therefore become impacted in small arterioles, causing ischaemia and further hypoxia. The abnormal haemoglobins may occur in combination with normal haemoglobin or with one another, producing a series of different haemoglobinopathies:

(1) *sickle-cell trait*: haemoglobin A with haemoglobin S (AS);
(2) *sickle-cell disease*: haemoglobin S with haemoglobin S (SS);
(3) *sickle-cell haemoglobin C disease*: haemoglobin S with haemoglobin C (SC);
(4) *sickle-cell thalassaemia*: the sickle gene inherited from one parent and the thalassaemia gene from the other (SThal).

The prevalence of different sickling haemoglobinopathies varies in different parts of the world. In the Afro-Caribbean population in the United States, sickle-cell trait is estimated to affect 8% of the population, sickle-cell disease 0.4%, and sickle-cell haemoglobin C disease 0.2%.

Although there may be ischaemic atrophy of the iris and vascular occlusion in the conjunctival vessels, the most important ocular complication from sickling haemoglobinopathies is retinopathy. Proliferative sickle retinopathy varies from mild retinopathy, with peripheral arteriolar occlusion and arterio-venous anastomosis, to the severe form, with neovascularization, vitreous haemorrhage, and potential traction retinal detachment. Ocular complications are most severe in SC and SThal haemoglobinopathies. Treatment for new retinal blood vessels includes peripheral panretinal photocoagulation in the early stages of the disease. If traction retinal detachment occurs, vitrectomy may be indicated.

EALES'S DISEASE

Eales's disease is a peripheral retinal periphlebitis of unknown cause, typically occurring in young, healthy adults aged 20–40 years. It is a diagnosis of exclusion, when all other potential causes of retinal periphlebitis have been considered and eliminated. Males are more commonly affected, in a ratio of 3:1. The presenting symptom is usually floaters or blurring of vision, attributable to recurrent vitreous haemorrhages. Severe cases may progress to proliferative retinopathy, with vitreous haemorrhage and traction retinal detachment. In the early stage, panretinal photocoagulation may be effective, but vitrectomy is required in cases of persistent vitreous haemorrhage and retinal detachment.

Papilloedema

Transient slight-to-severe obscurations of vision lasting a few seconds up to half a minute, and occurring irregularly a few times in a week to many times per day (half a dozen per hour), may be associated with moderate or severe degrees of papilloedema, even when the cause does not otherwise involve the visual pathway. See Fig. 7.5 and p. 125.

Chapter 8

Gradual Painless Loss of Vision

Gradual painless loss of vision is the commonest presenting symptom in ophthalmic practice, and therefore it is important to have a clear understanding of its differential diagnosis. As this is a problem particularly of the elderly population, more than one cause of gradual painless visual impairment may be present at one time, e.g. cataract and macular degeneration. This is consistent with the possible presence of two or more quite different diseases, especially in the elderly. 'Multiple pathology' is quite common in that age group.

The main causes of gradual painless loss of vision (see also p. 208) are

- cataract
- glaucoma (but field loss is usually peripheral, not central, i.e. visual acuity is unimpaired until late in the disease; see Chapter 5);
- macular degeneration;
- diabetic eye disease, see Chapter 10.

Other less common causes of gradual painless loss of vision, generally occurring in an earlier age group, are

- (high) myopia;
- retinal detachment;
- central serous retinopathy;
- peripheral retinal degenerations, e.g. retinitis pigmentosa;
- tobacco – alcohol amblyopia (rare);
- progressive corneal dystrophy, especially keratoconus;
- retinopathy of prematurity;
- AIDS retinopathy.

Cataract

A cataract is an opacity in the lens (see Figs 8.1 and 8.2). See p. 78 regarding maturity and hypermaturity of cataractous lenses. The symptoms vary considerably from patient to patient. A small opacity or opacities at the lens periphery will produce minor symptoms, if any, whereas a dense central lens opacity will produce very severe loss of vision, especially if it is posterior subcapsular. The lens is an avascular, translucent structure; its gradual hardening with increasing age causes presbyopia (see p. 20). Most cataracts seen in clinical practice occur in the elderly, although many of the elderly do not develop cataract. Risk factors are increasing age, vascular hypertension, myopia, smoking, high ethanol consumption, some diuretics and other drugs (especially systemic corticosteroids) and trauma. The position of the opacity in the lens determines the clinical category.

Nuclear cataract is in the central area of the lens i.e. the nucleus (Fig. 8.1).

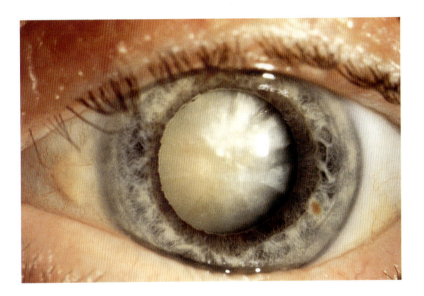

Fig. 8.1. Dense cataract. VA: perception of light (PL) with good projection. Some structure can still be seen: a peripheral cuneiform pattern (see also Fig. 8.2) plus central yellowish-brown nuclear opacity.

Posterior subcapsular cataract is usually sited immediately deep to the posterior lens capsule centrally. That site is in the optic axis of the eye near the nodal point, and therefore quite a small opacity may cause a disproportionate decrease in visual acuity.

Cortical cataracts are usually wedge-shaped opacities ('cuneiform cataracts') in the periphery of the lens cortex and progress slowly, seldom causing significant impairment of visual acuity, until eventually the central area of the lens is affected (Fig. 8.2).

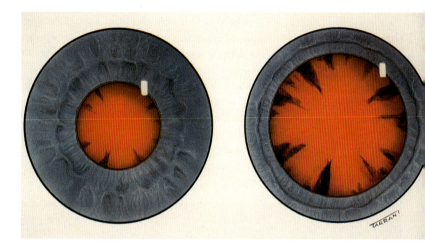

Fig. 8.2. Cuneiform (wedge-shaped) opacities, in the periphery of the eye lens, which are not initially disabling (VA 6/6 but with some glare in sunshine) and only slowly progressive. They are easier to see through a dilated pupil (picture on your right), and by looking through an ophthalmoscope (zero lens in peephole) from 0.33 or 0.5 m distance (or close up with + 10D lens), which elicits the red reflex to act as a contrasting background. With focal illumination (= close inspection with bright illuminating light only), the opacities are white.

Mixed cataracts are common, with some of the above, but cortical cataract tends to occur alone.

SYMPTOMS

The patient complains of a gradual decrease in visual acuity, usually over a period of months or years. One eye is usually more affected than the other. Glare in sunshine is frequently disabling.

SIGNS

The cardinal sign is an opacity in the lens, which is easily identified with the direct ophthalmoscope (p. 15) or focal illumination.

TREATMENT

The only really effective treatment at present for cataract is surgical removal of the lens, but the operation is deferred until the patient's standard of life is significantly affected by the cataract. In the meantime, a change in spectacles may alleviate some of the disability, e.g. stronger reading spectacles (with print held close to the eyes) and a good light. Some patients may tolerate significant decrease in visual acuity in both eyes, while to a very few others the earliest blurring of vision in one eye may be intolerable. As a very general rule, cataract extraction is performed in the worst eye when the vision in the better eye is 6/18 or less, although operation may be required at an earlier stage if there is a proportionately greater diminution of near vision, as may frequently occur with posterior subcapsular cataracts.

Surgical cataract extractions are of two main types, although there are many individual variants within each procedure. In both, an incision ('section') is made at the upper corneo-scleral junction (limbus) into the anterior chamber.

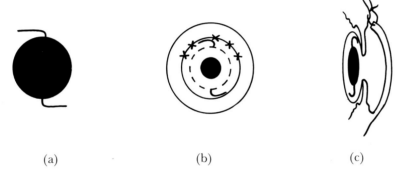

(a)   (b)   (c)

Fig. 8.3. (a) Intraocular lens (IOL) with two springy fixation-loops. (b) IOL in situ behind iris, dotted line indicating its edge, except in pupil area (black). Crosses represent five limbal sutures. (c) Vertical section of anterior segment of the eye showing lens (black oval) behind iris with loops in the 'capsular bag'. In this case, the surgeon has excised the anterior capsule from a little more than the pupil area, then removed the cataractous contents of the remaining capsule. Alternatively, the whole anterior capsule is removed so that the fixation-loops lie in the sulcus between the ciliary body and the base of the iris. (Note the loose suture at 12 o'clock, predisposing to iris prolapse and/or flat anterior chamber postoperatively!)

Extracapsular Cataract Extraction (ECCE) with Implantation of an Intraocular Lens (IOL)
This is at present the most popular tenchique, illustrated diagrammatically in Fig. 8.3, and should be seen being done in the operation theatre. An opening is made in the anterior lens capsule

through which the (hard) nucleus is removed. The nucleus may either be removed intact, or be disintegrated initially by ultrasound through a slim probe (phaco-emulsification) and then aspirated. The residual (soft) cortical lens matter is also aspirated, then an intraocular lens (Fig. 8.4) is usually implanted immediately behind the iris (supported posteriorly by the intact posterior lens capsule), after which the corneo-scleral wound of entry into the eyeball is sutured.

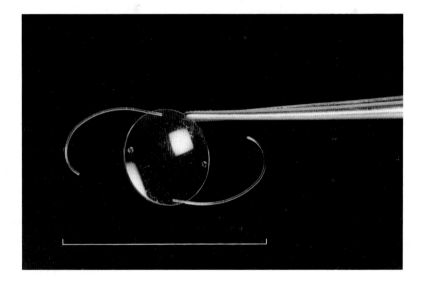

Fig. 8.4. An intraocular lens (IOL) currently in common use, for insertion just behind the plane of the iris, after removal of the cataractous contents of the lens capsule. See also Fig. 8.3. The clear plastic optic will occupy more than the pupil area. The springy loops will fixate the optic by resting in the equator of the capsular bag or (if the whole of the anterior lens capsule is removed) by resting in the sulcus between the ciliary body and the base of the iris. The optic is made of PMMA (polymethylmethacrylate) as for hard contact lenses, with hydroxyphenyl benzotriazole to absorb ultraviolet rays. In this particular lens the loops are also made of PMMA. Scale bar = 10 mm.

Intracapsular Cataract Extraction (ICCE)

This technique has become less popular with the advent of improved microsurgical operation techniques and of intraocular lenses. In this operation, the whole lens is removed, along with, and within, its capsule. This is usually facilitated by a cryoprobe, which freezes on to the surface of the lens, permitting the lens to be removed with minimal disturbance to the remainder of the ocular contents.

Aphakia

An eye without a lens (in the pupil aperture) is called an aphakic eye. It has a severe refractive error (hypermetropia) of about 10 dioptres, if the eye was emmetropic before operation. There are basically three methods by which this refractive error may be corrected: spectacle lens; contact lens (see p. 29 and Figs 3.7 and 3.8); and intraocular lens (IOL), usually inserted at the time of the cataract operation.

The positioning of a spectacle lens and a contact lens relative to the eye is straightforward, but the positioning of a lens within the eye (an intraocular lens) requires a little more explanation. An artificial plastic intraocular lens (IOL) may be placed in one of three positions:

- In the anterior chamber, anterior to the iris. This position is not ideal, as there is a significant risk of contact with the corneal endothelium, which is essential in pumping fluid out of the cornea; damage to it will cause corneal oedema and a need for corneal transplant. Some damage to the trabecular meshwork is also probable (see p. 52).
- In the plane of the pupil aperture, fixed to the iris by small loops in front of and behind the iris. This type of lens is seldom used nowadays, because of the high risk of damage to the corneal endothelium, as well as of iritis and displacement of the lens following pupillary dilation.
- In the posterior chamber (Figs 8.3 and 8.4). This is undoubtedly the most satisfactory position for an intraocular lens, and is physiologically in the same position as the natural lens that has been removed. It is also the safest position, away from fragile structures such as the cornea and the trabecular meshwork.

There is one simple rule that forms the basis for lens correction in the postoperative cataract patient: the greater the distance between the correcting lens and the eye, the greater the distortion of the image on the retina. In other words, a spectacle lens would cause greater distortion than a contact lens which, in turn, would cause more distortion than an intraocular lens in a given individual. In fact, a spectacle lens necessary to correct vision following cataract extraction increases the size of the image presented to the retina by up to one-third. In the case of a unilateral cataract (without an IOL) corrected by a spectacle lens, the retinal image in the operated eye is 20–35% larger than that in the unoperated eye. The visual system cannot fuse two such different images, so that a patient loses binocular vision after extraction of a unilateral cataract unless a contact lens is supplied or an intraocular lens is inserted. An alternative is for the patient to use only one eye, either the operated eye (corrected by a spectacle lens) or, more usually, the unoperated eye. The spectacle lens required following cataract extraction is very thick, which results in distortions (e.g. straight lines become curved), reduction in the peripheral field of vision, and impaired judgement of distance.

Contact lenses are discussed in Chapter 3, p. 29; see Figs 3.7 and 3.8. In high ametropia, e.g. aphakia (or high myopia), distortion with contact lenses is far less than with spectacles. Binocular vision is possible, as the increase in image size is only about 6%, which is within the tolerance of most people's visual systems. However, there are potentially serious complications with contact lenses, and elderly patients, possibly with arthritis, find contact lenses difficult or impossible to manage.

Intraocular lenses are the ideal optical method for correcting visual acuity. There are obviously potential complications of the more complex technique required, but in the hands of a skilled surgeon the small increase in the complication rate is acceptable.

Glaucoma

Glaucoma is discussed in detail in Chapter 5, and must always be excluded in cases of gradual painless loss of vision.

Macular Degeneration

APPLIED ANATOMY

The macula is the area (approximately 5 mm in diameter) enclosed by the superior and inferior temporal branches of the central retinal artery (Fig. 8.5). The *fovea* is an area of diameter 1.5 mm in the centre of the macula, and the *foveola*, a region consisting only of cones, is in the centre of the fovea. See Fig. 1.1. The highest concentration of photoreceptors (cones) occurs in the foveola, so that the fine acuity of central vision is dependent upon the integrity of this tiny area.

SYMPTOMS

The main symptom of macular disease is a gradual decrease in central visual acuity, usually bilateral, but often unequal. *The patient may also complain of distortion of images in the early stages.* The macula may be involved in several important disorders (diabetes mellitus, myopia, toxic maculopathies, especially chloroquine, and occasionally

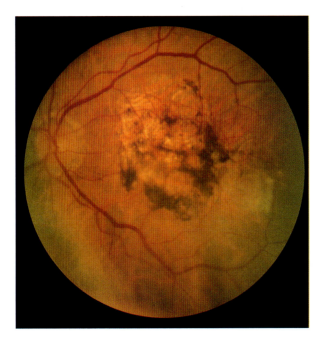

Fig. 8.5. Advanced senile ('age-related') macular degeneration, 'dry' type, causing a large central scotoma. VA: 'counting fingers' (CF) eccentrically. Almost the whole area between the superior and inferior temporal vessels is atrophic and pale, but obscured by large irregular areas of pigmentation. The normal optic disc is seen on the nasal side of the lesion, and does not show the usual temporal pallor of macular degeneration. In the earliest stages, the pigmentary disturbance is usually very slight and much more localized.

hypertension) but the commonest maculopathy is senile, or age-related, macular degeneration. It is subdivided clinically into 'non-exudative' or 'dry' and 'exudative' or 'wet'; the usual result of both types is progressive loss of visual acuity in both eyes, leading eventually to bilateral central scotomata, but with retained peripheral fields of vision. (Rare forms of macular degeneration, usually hereditary, can affect any younger age group.)

Non-exudative (Dry) Macular Degeneration

This is characterized by atrophy of the retinal receptors and underlying retinal pigment epithelium within the macula. The ophthalmoscopic appearance is usually of pigment clumping in the macular area, or occasionally a 'macular hole'. See Fig. 8.5.

There is no effective treatment for 'dry' macular degeneration, but central vision may be improved by magnification produced by various low-vision aids, e.g. hand magnifier for reading (or telescope for distance, which is not often successful).

Exudative (Wet) Macular Degeneration

This occurs when the retinal pigment epithelium detaches from Bruch's membrane, which separates choroid from retinal pigment epithelium, at the macula. It is often a consequence of creeping of fragile new blood vessels beneath the retinal pigment epithelium, which then leak plasma or rupture causing a haemorrhage. The haemorrhage beneath the retina often breaks through the neurosensory retina, causing a sudden loss of central vision. The haemorrhage gradually resolves, leaving a macular scar but no improvement in visual acuity.

Careful assessment of all macular degenerative conditions is essential to exclude slight elevation of the macular area, which may be an early sign of new vessels beneath the retina. If this is suspected, a fundus fluorescein angiogram is performed as an urgent procedure to demonstrate the position of subretinal new vessels. If new vessels are detected at an early stage and are not dangerously near the fovea, they may be destroyed by a laser beam, thereby preventing further loss of vision, although more new vessels may develop later and require repeat treatments. Unfortunately, the majority of patients present after the haemorrhage or leakage has already occurred in one eye, and it is therefore essential to assess the other eye carefully in these patients. Because exudative macular degeneration is treatable in the early stages, the patient should be warned to look for distortion in the centre of the field, e.g. straight vertical or horizontal lines develop a localized kink.

Once again, there is no effective treatment after the haemorrhage has occurred apart from low-vision aids as mentioned earlier. Many patients with macular degeneration that has destroyed 'reading vision' are terrified that their central scotomas (blind areas) will progress outwards to produce complete blindness. They are usually greatly encouraged to be told that this will not happen and that their peripheral fields will be retained; accordingly they will be able to walk around safely under most circumstances (navigating vision). It is also important to explain to patients that although they may have been placed on the blind or partially-sighted register (see p.8) this is a legal definition which enables the patient to obtain certain benefits to which they are entitled, and does *not* imply further loss of sight.

Diabetic Eye Disease

See Chapter 10. The commonest causes of visual loss in diabetics are retinopathy, cataracts and glaucoma.

(High) Myopia

Myopia (short-sightedness) is explained in Chapter 3, p. 25. In myopia, the rays of light entering the eye are focused at a point in front of the retina, usually because the axial length of the eyeball is abnormally great; occasionally the refractive power of the cornea and eye lens is stronger than that required for an eyeball of normal axial length.

Myopia may predispose the eye to potentially serious complications, but these tend to be associated specifically with high myopia, i.e. usually a refractive error of at least 7 dioptres, which obviously affects only a minority of myopes in the population.

Myopia predisposes to rhegmatogenous retinal detachment (due to retinal hole — see below), macular degeneration (see p. 112), open angle glaucoma (see p. 72) and cataract (see p. 106). Rhegmatogenous retinal detachment (see below) and the macular degeneration associated with myopia can be partly explained by stretching of the retina. The retina was originally designed to line an eyeball of about 24 mm in axial length, but the myopic eyeball starts to grow unusually large from around 7 years of age. By the age of 18 years or so, the axial length may reach as much as 30 mm or even more, so that the retina is abnormally thin with some degenerative changes, mainly anteriorly and at the posterior pole.

Retinal Detachment

Detachment of the retina describes the situation when the neurosensory retina becomes separated from the underlying pigment epithelium (Fig. 1.2 and pp. 2 and 3). There are four fundamental categories of retinal detachment, based upon the pathological mechanisms involved.

Rhegmatogenous Detachment (Break-Caused or Tear-caused).
This accounts for the majority of cases. Most cases of retinal detachment are caused by a tear in the retina, usually superiorly (Fig. 8.6). The tear is produced as follows. First, cavities appear in the vitreous of the ageing or aphakic or myopic eye so that the vitreous collapses and detaches from the retina. Some vitreous floaters occur at this stage but no other

significant symptoms are produced in this very common situation. The vitreous detaches from the retina from behind forwards until, far anteriorly, in a few eyes, the vitreous tugs on a spot or spots of vitreo-retinal fibrotic adhesions (caused by previous peripheral retinal degenerative changes). Either a round hole results, if the vitreous pulls off a 'plug' of retina, or a 'horseshoe' or 'arrowhead' tear is produced, always with its apex pointing posteriorly towards the disc. Through that hole or tear seeps more and more of the fluid surrounding the collapsed vitreous to cause a retinal detachment (which we should, strictly call an intraretinal separation, just as we should strictly replace 'subretinal fluid' by 'intraretinal fluid'; see pp. 2 and 3).

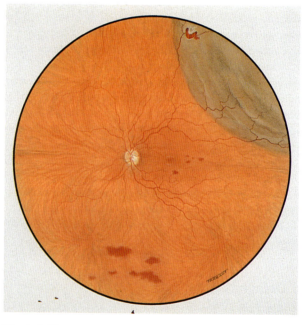

Fig. 8.6. Horse-shoe or arrowhead tear with *retinal* detachment supero-temporally in a – 5D myopic eye in a man aged 55 years. VAL 6/6 with spectacles, but the presenting symptoms a week previously were a *sudden* shower of floaters, due to haemorrhage from the retinal vessel ruptured when the tear/hole occurred — blotches of red blood cells are still visible in the lower vitreous. Three to four days previously, a 'black blob' towards the point of the nose appeared, corresponding to the supero-temporal area of retinal detachment which has resulted from seepage of fluid surrounding the collapsed vitreous through the hole; gravity causes the accumulating fluid to spread downwards as shown. See also Figs 8.7 and 8.8.

In addition to myopia, other predisposing factors are age (over, say, 60 years), trauma, aphakia, retinal neovascularization, e.g. in diabetics (see below) and, of course, a previous history of retinal detachment in the same eye (successfully treated previously) or the other eye.

Traction Detachment (Less Common)
In traction retinal detachment, contraction of quite dense fibrous bands within the vitreous pulls the neurosensory retina from the retinal pigment epithelium. A hole may also be pulled off the retina as a result of contraction of bands. By far the commonest cause is diabetes mellitus (see Chapter 10).

'Solid' Retinal Detachment (Rare)
The retina is detached by a solid mass behind the retina, e.g. malignant choroidal melanoma, or metastases in the choroid from a distant primary neoplasm, especially of breast.

Exudative Detachment
Under this rather unsatisfactory general heading, we would mention the (small) area of retinal detachment inferiorly that can occur, usually in both eyes, in hypoproteinaemia or dysproteinaemia, the nephrotic syndrome and toxaemia of pregnancy. The subretinal fluid is analogous to the oedema elsewhere characteristic of these conditions. It accumulates in the subretinal or, strictly, intraretinal potential space, into which also fluid seeps in rhegmatogenous detachments. Both remind us of the embryological development of the retina (pp. 2 and 3).

SYMPTOMS

The classical symptoms of rhegmatogenous retinal detachment are

- sudden onset of 'flashing lights' (photopsiae), because the vitreous 'tugs' on the retina;
- sudden shower of 'floaters' in one eye, if a retinal blood vessel is ruptured in the process of tear formation (see Fig. 8.6); occasionally the vitreous chamber is completely filled with blood;
- gradually increasing field defect, often described as a 'curtain' or 'black cloud', moving from below upwards.

These symptoms should always be considered as serious and the patient *immediately* referred to an ophthalmic department for *urgent* assessment, especially if he is a myope. Whilst retinal detachment is a surgical emergency, it is nevertheless a relatively uncommon condition in the general population.

SIGNS

- Retinal detachment is most appropriately assessed by binocular indirect ophthalmoscopy, but the diagnosis can certainly be made using the (uniocular) direct ophthalmoscope, providing a careful examination of the peripheral retina is performed.
- A widely dilated pupil is neccesary for adequate examination (see p. 11). Note that these eyes are usually myopic and have deep anterior chambers, which means that there is a quite negligible risk of producing acute closed-angle glaucoma by mydriatics (p. 70).
- The typical appearance of a rhegmatogenous detachment is a greyish convex membrane (retina) 'ballooning' into the vitreous, usually from above, and undulating to some extent with movements of the head or eye. Retinal vessels appear black and are tortuous. See Fig. 8.6.

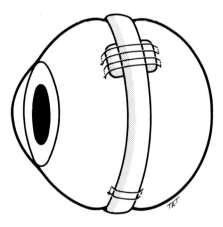

Fig. 8.7. Diagram of operation for the retinal detachment shown in Figs 8.6 and 8.8. A silicone band encircles and slightly constricts the equatorial plane of the eyeball, to relieve traction by vitreous bands and to help maintain the localized indentation of the plomb sutured to the surface of the sclera over the retinal hole. Fig. 8.8 shows the ophthalmoscopic view after the operation. Tethering sutures are also placed on the nasal side of the eyeball.

TREATMENT

Treatment depends on the stage at which the diagnosis is made. If only a retinal hole is present, light coagulation by laser can 'spot-weld' the retina around the hole, thereby preventing the seepage of fluid through the hole that detaches the retina. Usually, however, the retina is detached and an operation is required. See Figs 8.6, 8.7 and 8.8. An area of 'sticky' choroiditis is produced by a freezing cryoprobe applied to the outer surface of the sclera in the region to which the retinal hole is

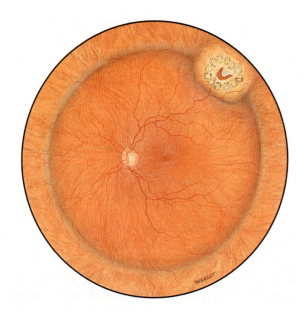

Fig. 8.8. Cryopexy with a plomb and encircling band has 'cured' the *retinal* detachment shown in Fig. 8.6. See also Fig. 8.7. A cryoprobe has been applied to the outer surface of the sclera over the hole-bearing area of the retina to produce a mild choroiditis with a 'sticky' exudate. A plomb is sutured to the surface of the sclera over the hole to form the plateau, obvious in the picture, on which that area of retina will rest. Often release of subretinal fluid is also required by an incision through sclera and choroid over the detached area. Thus the retina sinks back on to its bed, and the retina around the hole is sealed off by the sticky, later pale, atrophic choroid. The fainter evidence of a raised area of retina all round the equatorial region results from an encircling band whose function is (a) to maintain pressure on the plomb and therefore retain the raised plateau and (b) to reduce the equatorial diameter of the eyeball, thereby reducing 'vitreous traction', and the risk of recurrence of hole-formation and retinal detachment.

estimated to correspond. Subretinal fluid is usually evacuated by an incision through sclera and choroid, thereby 'floating' the retina back towards its bed. To help the hole-bearing area of retina to settle on to the now sticky, mildly inflamed choroid, a silicone (sponge) 'plomb' is sutured tightly to the surface of the sclera over the hole thus pushing the wall of the eyeball towards the retinal hole; this process is often aided by placing an encircling band of silicone around the eyeball, and ensuring that the plomb is underneath the band. For the same purpose, a large bubble of air, or silicone oil in some circumstances, may be injected into the vitreous cavity.

In the case of traction detachment, vitrectomy may be necessary (see p. 144).

Central Serous Retinopathy

Central serous retinopathy presents with a reasonably slow onset (days) of a *slight* decrease of visual acuity in one eye to, say, 6/9 or 6/12, usually in males aged between 20 and 45 years. It is caused by a defect in the retinal pigment epithelium, whereby fluid passes through the epithelium and elevates the neurosensory retina, usually at the macula. Objects seen by the affected eye look smaller (micropsia) than objects from the normal eye because retinal cones are spread apart by the macular oedema. Most cases resolve within a few months, often without treatment, but laser photocoagulation of the defect in the pigment epithelium may be necessary in a very small proportion of cases.

Peripheral Retinal Degeneration

The most important peripheral retinal degeneration is retinitis pigmentosa, which is discussed in Chapter 16, p. 199. See Fig. 16.1.

Tobacco–Alcohol Amblyopia

Tobacco–alcohol amblyopia is characterized by bilateral reduction of central visual acuity, associated with impairment of colour vision 'in the presence of a normal ocular examination', occurring in subjects with excessive tobacco and/or alcohol intake. Predisposing factors are poor diet, malnutrition, partial gastrectomy or gastro-enterostomy, malabsorption and diabetes. Some evidence incriminates chronic cyanide poisoning (possibly from insecticides sprayed onto tobacco plants), which can be detoxicated by injections of large doses of hydroxocobalamin. Probably a similar disease is 'tropical amblyopia' due to eating cassava. The patient should be advised to stop smoking, and drinking alcohol, and adopt a well-balanced diet. Gradual improvement in vision usually accompanies the change in lifestyle, although some visual impairment may be permanent in some patients.

Progressive Corneal Dystrophy: Corneal Grafts

A large variety of rare hereditary progressive corneal degenerations exists with patchy opacification specific for each condition. All are avascular. Keratoconus is the least uncommon; the central area of the cornea thins and bulges forwards: the probable cause is autosomal recessive genes (see also p. 26). When and if spectacles, then contact lenses, fail to achieve adequate improvement in vision, a corneal graft is required (Fig. 8.9).

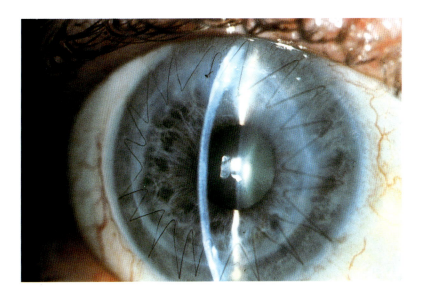

Fig. 8.9. A slit-lamp photograph of a full-thickness (penetrating) corneal graft (keratoplasty). The continuous monofilament nylon suture is producing no inflammatory reaction.

The ideal candidate for corneal graft has a bilateral severe disturbance of the central cornea, non-vascularized (e.g. keratoconus), that cannot be improved significantly enough in the better eye by spectacles or contact lenses. The worst situation is bilateral heavily scarred, vascularized corneae, e.g. following a lime burn: even if a technically satisfactory operation can be done, the presence of lymphatics accompanying the blood vessels produces a very high risk of a host-versus-graft reaction with opacification and vascularization of the donor disc. See Fig. 8.9.

By far the commonest technique is to trephine a 5, 6 or 7 mm diameter full-thickness disc from the central cornea of a healthy donor eye (ideally matched with the recipient's HLA profile, especially if the cornea is vascularized) and suture it into the same size of disc trephined from the recipient's eye. Very occasionally a lamellar (i.e. partial-thickness) corneal graft is possible if the opacification of the cornea is only superficial.

Retinopathy Of Prematurity

During late intrauterine life, retinal vessels grow in response to the demand for oxygen by the developing, thickening retina. In premature low-birth-weight babies, prolonged exposure to high levels of oxygen in their incubators produces high levels of tissue oxygen (in the case of the retina, derived from the choroidal circulation) so that growth of the retinal vessels ceases. By the time the extra breathed oxygen is withdrawn, the retina has developed further so that its oxygen needs have increased considerably. The retinal blood vessels respond by excessive proliferation into the retina, and also into the vitreous. These abnormal intravitreous vessels carry a scaffolding of fibrous tissue which later contracts and causes progressive retinal detachment. In severe cases, a white mass of fibrous tissue and retina lies behind the lens — 'retrolental fibroplasia' is the old name for the tragic end-stage of this iatrogenic disease.

Its frequency has diminished considerably as premature babies are now given the minimum duration and concentration of oxygen, and ophthalmoscopic monitoring is used to detect the earliest stages of peripheral retinal arterio-venous shunt vessels (stimulated by angiogenic products from immature ischaemic retina). When these are observed, good results can be achieved by cryotherapy via a probe applied to the scleral surface over, or by laser through the pupil to, the far peripheral retina. However, the child will have a long-term predisposition to myopia, retinal detachment and, surprisingly, closed-angle glaucoma.

AIDS Retinopathy

Transient small cottonwool spots in the retina are common in acquired immune deficiency syndrome (AIDS). Much more sinister and sight-threatening are the large, confluent snowballs of opportunistic metastatic infections, especially by cytomegalovirus. Intravitreous injections of antibiotic may be part of the treatment strategy.

Chapter 9

Neuro-ophthalmology

The ophthalmologist must remain a general physician and surgeon to an important extent; his involvement in neurology has even greater relevance. Conversely, the neurologist must be significantly involved in ophthalmology. For the non-specialist some knowledge of neuro-ophthalmology is a very useful firm basis from which to view neurology as a whole.

This superspecialty will be presented anatomically but only the common conditions can be mentioned. Investigations that are the province of the neurologist have been omitted.

Optic Nerve

Multiple or disseminated sclerosis (MS or DS) often presents in the late 'teens or twenties with a 'retrobulbar neuritis' in which a plaque of demyelination causes progressive painless loss of central vision (central scotoma) over a period of around a week. The adage 'the patient and the ophthalmologist see nothing' emphasizes the normal fundus appearances in spite of a visual acuity of less than 6/60. If the plaque is at the apex of the orbit, pain on looking up is characteristic because the origin of the superior rectus muscle pulls on the inflamed area of the optic nerve.

Very rarely, the plaque may be at or just behind the optic disc, hence 'papillitis' which is easily recognized ophthalmoscopically as a volcanic eruption — splashes of haemorrhage and exudate on, and near, a papilloedematous disc; other causes of papillitis are very, very rare. The visual acuity is poor (compare papilloedema due to raised intracranial pressure, in which visual acuity is usually normal). Although central retinal vein occlusion produces a rather similar ophthalmoscopic picture (Figs 7.2 and 7.3), it is very rare in the late 'teens or twenties.

Typically the visual acuity returns to normal in 3–5 weeks, but occasionally permanent optic atrophy with poor vision ensues. 'Temporal pallor' of the optic disc is said to be common in MS but it is common in 'normal' eyes especially if myopic; the commonest cause of temporal pallor in an eye clinic is actually macular degeneration.

Provided that there are no other neurological signs or symptoms of MS when retrobulbar neuritis occurs, *almost 50% of patients will probably escape any other manifestations of the disease.* The other 50% will probably develop progressive MS; around one-third of that 50% will probably suffer restricted activity by the end of 10 years. The authors usually take the opportunity diplomatically to tell the patient early in the episode that there is an inflammation of the optic nerve behind the eye of which the cause is unknown, but that it almost invariably recovers. Depending on age and circumstances, the authors advise that unnecessary stress, such as pregnancy or ambitious career ventures, should be avoided for about four years; by the end of such a recurrence-free period, following an episode of retrobulbar neuritis with no other symptoms or signs, the prognosis improves considerably.

Remarkably often, the patients sooner or later can attach the diagnosis 'MS' to their condition. However, it must be emphasized that, as the name suggests, a diagnosis of multiple sclerosis requires at least two characteristic episodes of neurological deficit, separated in time and site. Accordingly, as emphasized above, a single episode of retrobulbar neuritis does not necessarily imply progressive multiple sclerosis, which term is probably best not volunteered to the patient in order to avoid unnecessary distress.

Optic atrophy is never a diagnosis: its cause has to be specified. A pale optic disc, usually with poor visual acuity and a reduced field of vision, can have many local causes, e.g. occlusion of the central retinal artery (p. 93) or (in giant cell arteritis) of the blood supply to the anterior optic nerve (p. 101), but the commonest is probably the special case of glaucoma in which the atrophy is associated with pathological cupping of the disc (Fig. 5.3a, b). Head injury is another cause, easily diagnosed from the history; a fracture of the skull may well not be present. Multiple sclerosis has been mentioned as one cause of optic atrophy in the previous section. Although rare, an intracranial space-occupying lesion is an important differential diagnosis: usually there are other signs and symptoms, of which anosmia is easily overlooked.

Papilloedema can easily be mistakenly diagnosed (see Fig. 7.5) in the following circumstances.

- In a hypermetropic (i.e. small) eye in which retinal nerve fibres are crowded together, and so raised, as they escape through a small optic disc: the absence of the optic cup also misleads.
- When drusen are present in the disc, but a glinting crystalline spot or two can usually be seen ophthalmoscopically at one or more points in a 'lumpy' disc.
- When refractive errors, especially astigmatism, or opacities in the

media, particularly slight corneal opacities, produce blurring of the disc margins for the ophthalmoscopist, and blurred vision for the patient.

These should be considered if the history or other clinical signs are not consistent with raised intracranial pressure.

The clinical characteristics of papilloedema due to raised intracranial pressure are easily understood from the known mechanism. See Fig. 7.5. The raised intracranial pressure is transmitted all the way down the extension of the subarachnoid space that envelops the whole of the optic nerve. Back-pressure is exerted on the circulation at the optic disc, hence:

- absence of spontaneous venous pulsation of the central retinal vein on ophthalmoscopy;
- hyperaemia of the disc;
- small splinter haemorrhages on the disc surface (very, very characteristic);
- accumulation of tissue fluid (oedema).

Blockage at the disc of axoplasmic flow in the axons of the retinal ganglion cells contributes significantly to the swelling. In the early stages, it may be difficult to detect the slight blurring of the disc margin superiorly and inferiorly at first, then all round. In severe cases, the oedematous papilla may be pushed so far into the vitreous that the ophthalmoscopist can utilize parallax (p. 13 and Fig. 2.6) between its tip and the retina: by moving his head-plus-ophthalmoscope slightly, he can see that tip moving in relation to the background retina.

An intravenous injection of fluorescein immediately followed by fundus photography through filters is rarely required to assist in the diagnosis: leakage of fluid from the hyperaemic circulation at the disc is characteristic.

Usually the visual acuity is normal. It is usually bilateral but often asymmetrical; especially in the early stages, one disc may even be normal. When papilloedema is due to raised intracranial pressure, two other members of the classic triad of papilloedema, headache and vomiting, may also be present, often with other signs and symptoms. If accelerated hypertension is the cause, usually in a young adult, hypertensive retinopathy is usually also obvious; anyway, the blood pressure is greatly raised.

The papilloedema of central retinal vein occlusion is associated with widespread splotches of large haemorrhages and some exudates *all over the fundus*; it is usually unilateral and the affected eye has poor visual acuity. See Figs 7.2 and 7.3.

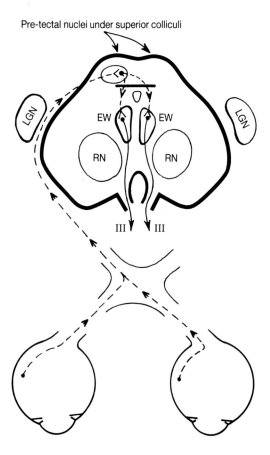

Pre-tectal nuclei under superior colliculi

Fig. 9.1. Pupillary-light reflex. Diagrammatic section through mid-brain and anterior visual pathway including chiasma. EW = Edinger – Westphal nucleus. RN = red nucleus. LGN = lateral geniculate nucleus. III = third cranial or oculomotor nerve. Dotted lines show afferent pathways, the continuous lines (III) show the efferent paths. Solid horizontal bar above the cerebral aqueduct of Sylvius (𝖢) indicates probable site of the lesion in the Argyll–Robertson pupil (p.129). For simplicity, the mirror-image pathways on the other side have been omitted. See text for details, and for the near reflex.

Normal Pupil Reactions

The light reflex is a pupil contraction in both eyes when a light is shone into one eye. It is called the 'direct light reflex' in the stimulated eye and the 'consensual light reflex' in the other eye. When that test gives a normal result, the following neural pathway is intact (see Fig. 9.1): retina, optic nerve, optic tract until a bundle of fibres separates off before the geniculate body; that bundle passes to the region of the superior colliculi on both sides (relay) from which connections pass to the Edinger–Westphal parts of *both* oculomotor (III) nuclei (relay); the efferent pathway then traverses both oculomotor nerves into the orbits and their branches to the ciliary ganglions from which short ciliary branches pass forwards to pierce the sclera around the optic nerves and so reach the ciliary body and iris. The reflex contraction of the pupil reduces the amount of light reaching the retina.

The near reflex also starts from the retina and eventually causes contraction of the pupils of both eyes, in association with both accommodation and convergence. The arc is different from that of the light reflex (Fig. 9.1): retina and optic nerve are common, but the afferent limb continues to the lateral geniculate body. Surprisingly, there is doubt about the next part of the arc, which may proceed to the calcarine (occipital) cortex as part of the visual pathway, then to the nearby peristriate area. From there, a cortico-tectal pathway carries impulses to the Edinger–Westphal nuclei. These nuclei are well-accepted relay stations which then use the IIIrd nerves to reach both medial recti (for convergence) and, via the ciliary ganglia, the sphincter muscles of both pupils and both ciliary muscles (for accommodation). There is also a shorter reflex arc that independently can cause, or contribute reinforcement to, the near pupil reflex: it arises in proprioceptive endings in the medial recti, passes up both Vth or IIIrd nerves and utilizes the same efferent pathway from the Edinger – Westphal nuclei. Contraction of the pupils, like that of the iris diaphragm of a camera, increases the depth of focus.

Abnormal Pupils and Pupil Reactions

In an eye clinic the commonest causes are probably drugs that dilate the pupils (mydriatics), e.g. atropine, homatropine, tropicamide and cyclopentolate (which paralyse the sphincter of the pupil under parasympathetic control) or adrenaline and phenylephrine (which stimulate the dilator pupillae, under sympathetic control), or drugs that constrict the pupil (miotics), e.g. pilocarpine and occasionally physostigmine (eserine). Diseases or injuries, including operations that excise or distort the iris or cause the pupil or the iris to be fibrosed to lens or cornea, are also common, e.g. iridocyclitis, perforating wounds of cornea, including drainage operations for glaucoma and cataract extractions.

Do NOT use mydriatics or miotics if the state of the pupil is important for diagnosis and management, e.g. especially in cases of head injury or coma. Unilateral pupillary enlargement, or fixed dilated pupil, may be an early sign of pressure on the third cranial nerve by a temporal lobe herniating through the tentorial hiatus: important causes are supratentorial space-occupying lesions including tumour and ruptured aneurysm of the internal carotid. Pupils become smaller with increasing age. Very small pupils suggest pontine haemorrhage or morphine poisoning, especially in a comatose patient.

An *'afferent pupil defect'* means an absent response on that side to light shone into a completely blind eye (no perception of light) or a poor response ('relative afferent pupil defect') in an eye with reduced sensitivity to light from any cause, e.g. dense cataract, partial optic atrophy. Even if the other eye has good vision, its consensual pupillary light response will also be absent or poor, respectively. However, a light shone into a normal eye will produce pupil constriction in the other eye (as well as on the stimulated side) whether the latter is blind or sees poorly. An afferent pupil defect may exist in both eyes, of course.

The Argyll–Robertson pupils, of great neurological interest, are rarely seen nowadays because neurosyphilis is so uncommon. They are typically bilateral, usually small, and irregular, and fail to react to light directly and consensually but, very surprisingly, react briskly for near vision; the condition occurs mainly in men over 40 years. Mydriatics are ineffective. The lesion is probably between the pre-tectal nucleus and the oculo-motor (IIIrd) nucleus where it can block the pupil's light reflex, direct and consensual, but leave intact the near reflex. See Fig. 9.1. The knee and ankle jerks are absent.

The tonic (Holmes–Adie or Adie) pupil is much more common and important, and cannot be confused with the Argyll–Robertson pupil with which, however, it shares — very surprisingly — the absent (or very slow) response to light, direct and consensual, the brisk contraction for near (accommodation and convergence) and, amazingly, the frequent absence of the knee and ankle jerks. In contrast to the Argyll–Robertson pupil, the Holmes–Adie pupil affects usually young women, is usually unilateral and is dilated. The differential diagnosis is mainly accidental contamination by a mydriatic; recovery in a few days confirms that possibility, but a history of contact is usually available. A rare variant is a brisk light reaction and an absent or slow near reflex.

The patient can be reassured on the clinical findings that this curiosity does not imply any future CNS or other disease. The cause is unknown but pathological changes have been found in the ciliary ganglion in the orbit.

Horner's syndrome results from a lesion of the sympathetic pathway, almost always unilateral. It consists of

- a small pupil;
- slight ptosis;
- (only in lesions proximal to the superior cervical ganglion) absence of sweating of the skin of the face (plus head, arm and upper trunk if the lesion is within the CNS or spinal cord).

The site of the lesion is often difficult to locate in the long sympathetic nerve supply to, respectively,

- the dilator muscle of the pupil;
- Müller's muscle (which originates from the underside of the aponeurosis at the anterior end of the levator muscle of the upper lid, and inserts into the upper border of the tarsal plate in the upper lid);
- sweat glands.

The sympathetic pathway extends from the region of the thalamus, down the brainstem and cervical spinal cord to the T1 segment, at which it passes outwards to the lowest cervical sympathic ganglion then upwards through the whole sympathetic chain in the neck to form the sympathetic plexus surrounding the internal carotid artery before it enters the skull. That artery's branches then carry sympathetic innervation to the structures listed above, and to others.

The syndrome often occurs in isolation. Many cases are congential. A vascular cause is usually suspected in an older patient. Sometimes a 'Pancoast tumor' is incriminated, i.e. an apical bronchial carcinoma which has spread to the lowest cervical ganglion and which may also cause a T1 lesion.

Visual Field Defects

See Fig. 9.2. For methods of examination, see pp. 8 and 63, and Figs 2.3 and 5.11.

Pre-chiasmal (Optic Nerve) Lesions
A complete lesion of an optic nerve, e.g. injury or neoplasm, will produce complete blindness (no perception of light) on that side. A large

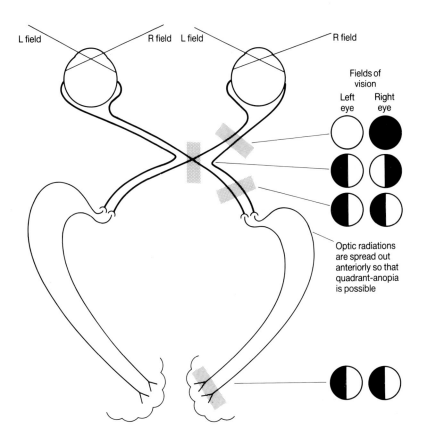

Fig. 9.2. A horizontal section through the brain at the level of the eyes shows the optic sensory pathways to the occipital (visual) cortex. Both eyes have a wide field of vision because the retina lines most of a sphere. Note that objects on the *left* produce images on the *right* halves of *both* retinae, while objects on the *right* produce images on the *left* halves of *both* retinae.

A lesion of the right optic *nerve* causes loss of the whole field in that eye with no effect on the left eye. A mid-line *chiasmal* lesion causes the classic bitemporal hemianopia. A lesion of the optic *tract* or, much more posteriorly, the occipital cortex produces a contralateral hemianopia with a sharp vertical edge. Because the optic radiations spread out in the temporal lobe as they circumvent the inferior horn of the lateral ventricle, a lesion there produces an irregular-edged, though still homonymous, defect in the contralateral field: a quadrantic defect is possible but is usually not exact, i.e. the scotoma may be greater than or less than a quarter of the field.

variety of patterns of *unilateral* field loss can be produced by partial lesions of one optic nerve, but the most characteristic is a central scotoma. Conversely, a pattern of bilaterally symmetrical field loss inexplicable by chiasmal or post-chiasmal lesions (see below) is usually due to bilateral retinal or optic nerve disease, e.g. the bilateral central scotoma of macular degeneration (p. 112), the arcuate and binasal defects of glaucoma (pp. 73 and 74).

Chiasmal Lesions: Bitemporal Hemianopia
(Hemianopia means the absence of vision in one half-field, usually to right or left of an imaginary vertical line down the centre of the field, passing through fixation.) The bitemporal hemianopia associated with an enlarged pituitary gland in an adult (an eosinophil adenoma in acromegaly, or a chromophobe adenoma) is well known, but in a child a suprasellar cyst may be the explanation. More generally, a mid-line lesion of the optic chiasma will interrupt the fibres from the nasal halves of both right and left retinae, hence the diagnostic pattern of field loss (see Fig. 9.2). Sometimes a mid-line pituitary neoplasm will extend into one or eventually both optic nerves to convert a temporal hemianopia on that side into complete blindness in that eye or eventually blindness in both eyes. Note that the vertical dividing line between nasal and temporal retinal receptors passes through the fovea centralis, not the optic disc. In albino animals, including humans, a variable proportion of axons from *temporal* ganglion cells cross over at the chiasma, as well as all the nasal fibres of course.

Post-chiasmal Lesions: Hemianopia and Quadrantanopia
The exact pattern of field loss in lesions posterior to the chiasma can be very useful in locating accurately the site of a neurological lesion. All have a homonymous ('the same side') property, i.e. the same *field* (right or left) is affected in *both* eyes. See Fig. 9.2. A complete homonymous hemianopia suggests a lesion of one occipital cortex, usually vascular. (Always test the field of vision, at least to confrontation, in the hemiplegic or 'C.V.A.' patient: it is easy to miss a hemianopia.) A less common cause is a lesion of one optic tract. A homonymous defect in one quadrant only, or less than a quadrant, or more than a quadrant (but not a complete hemianopia) is more characteristic of a temporal lobe lesion where the fibres in the optic radiations are more spread out (compare those in the tracts).

Because of involvement of the nearby parieto-occipital cortex, an occipital lesion producing hemianopia may also cause alexia (inability to recognize letters). The latter indicates a lesion of the dominant hemisphere, i.e. the left in a right-handed person. It may occur without hemianopia.

'Cortical blindness', which may be an isolated lesion, is usually due to an embolus or thrombosis at the point where the basilar artery divides into posterior cerebral arteries. Both occipital cortices cease to function. *Normal pupillary light reflexes are preserved.* That patient may well be less aware of blindness than is someone with bilateral eye disease.

Diplopia and Extraocular Muscle Paralysis

Diplopia (double vision) describes the situation in which two separate, usually quite clear, images are seen by the patient. It is usually binocular, i.e. due to a misalignment of the visual axes, and often the result of a nerve defect. However, uniocular 'diplopia' must be carefully differentiated, as follows.

Uniocular Diplopia
Sometimes a patient with unilateral cataract or slight corneal opacity will present with a complaint of double vision, which is accurate enough if a second (blurred) image seems to be more prominent than overall blurring. To eliminate that possibility, an early question to the patient is 'Does the double vision disappear if you shut the right eye' and '. . . left eye?' The answer 'yes' to both of these questions indicates 'binocular diplopia' whereas if the 'diplopia' remains in one eye when the other is closed, 'uniocular diplopia' is present and hence a search for cataract, etc. must be made. 'Uniocular diplopia' may affect each eye separately, of course.

Binocular Diplopia
The history can take the observer far along the road to identifying the muscle or nerve involved. Are the images side by side or one above the other? Is one image tilted? If the diplopia is horizontal (without tilt), an abducent (VIth) nerve lesion is likely, especially if the images are separated more in the right or left direction of gaze. See Fig. 4.5. Note that the separation of the diplopic images is maximal in the direction of action of the affected muscle. Vertical diplopia without (obvious) tilt of an image suggests involvement of a superior or inferior rectus (a 'vertical rectus'). An obvious tilt in one image suggests a IVth nerve or superior oblique muscle lesion because that muscle wheel-rotates the eyeball inwards as well as turning it to point downwards when the eye is also adducted towards the nose. See Fig. 4.6. A complete IIIrd (oculomotor) nerve lesion does not produce diplopia — because of complete ptosis! When the drooped eyelid is raised, the eyeball is seen to be

turned outwards by the intact lateral rectus muscle; the only other movement possible is wheel-rotation inwards of the upper eyeball (watch the iris at 12 o'clock) as a result of retained superior oblique function: watch a site on the iris while asking the patient to look down and to the opposite side.

Elucidation of the lesion of a muscle or nerve responsible for diplopia is made rather difficult because the lesion is usually incomplete, so that the action of a muscle is merely weakened (paresis) rather than completely abolished (paralysed). Even slight weakness causes diplopia that is immediately obvious and troublesome to the patient so that he consults his doctor usually immediately. *Impairment of movement may well not be obvious to the clinician scrutinizing such a patient's ocular movements.* Accordingly, the ophthalmologist often resorts to the Hess or Lees screen to identify the weak movement: the student should see these in the orthoptic department.

The Hess screen consists of, essentially, red dots at four corners of a square, with one also placed in the centre of each side of the square, on a black background. The patient wears a red goggle over his right eye and a green goggle over his left. The patient is asked to place a green spot of light from a torch on each red dot in turn. The observer plots on a chart the site of these 'green points'. In directions where the visual axes are unaffected, the green and red points coincide; elsewhere, the difference will be revealing, e.g. if a left lateral rectus is malfunctioning, on the left side of the chart, the green light will be placed at points short of the red points.

Spot diagnoses are often possible.

- A recent diplopia in a young adult with no other symptoms suggests multiple sclerosis; if so, it will recover in 3–4 weeks.
- In the elderly, a sudden paresis of an extra-ocular muscle also usually clears up in a few weeks (6–7 in this case) and is attributed rather vaguely to a 'vascular' cause (presumably atherosclerosis, hypertension or diabetes mellitus).

In both cases, of course, the differential diagnosis includes an intracranial neoplasm (see p. 137).

Diplopia in one direction of gaze due to a selective paralysis of a medial rectus muscle along with nystagmoid jerks of the lateral rectus on the other side clearly indicates an 'internuclear ophthalmoplegia'. A lesion of the anterior end of, say, the left medial longitudinal bundle (hence internuclear) will interrupt impulses to the medial rectus on that side when the fronto-motor eye field is sending messages to contract to both that medial rectus and to the lateral rectus on the right side. Although impulses to the right lateral rectus are getting through, the brain is recurrently sending reinforcing impulses to the unresponsive left medial rectus, hence the nystagmoid jerks by the lateral rectus muscle on the right side. In a young adult, the diagnosis is almost certain to be multiple sclerosis, while the elderly patient probably has a 'vascular lesion'.

The sudden onset of diplopia and headache suggests an intracranial aneurysm.

When 'spot' diagnoses have failed, and there is no history of injury, a systematic approach may be helpful, starting anteriorly.

- Orbital lesions are usually obvious because there is proptosis and/or redness of one or both eyes, e.g. especially in dysthyroid eye disease; muscles and fat are infiltrated with inflammatory autoimmune lymphocytes, followed eventually by fibroblasts. Neoplasms are rarities, primary or secondary (e.g. blood-borne metastases from carcinoma of breast or bronchus or local spread from tumours of sinus, pharynx, etc.).

- The neuromuscular junction should be specifically considered lest myasthenia gravis be missed. The onset may be quite sudden and unilateral. A Tensilon test is usually positive.

- Muscular lesions, i.e. a muscular dystrophy, sometimes purely of the extraocular muscles, will be the usual explanation for immobility of both eyes (diplopia seldom occurs): the patient will move his head when ocular movements are tested. Although 'senile ptosis' is to some extent physiological, a breakdown of the insertion of the levator palpebrae superioris into the upper tarsal plate often explains severe cases.

- Nerve lesions have been mainly considered in the previous section of this chapter.

- Gaze palsies due to supranuclear lesions are mentioned on p. 49.

Headache

Unfortunately, there is a widespread belief that headaches are often due to refractive errors and will be cured by appropriate spectacles. That is quite uncommon and will usually be excluded by a careful history of site, original time of onset, duration of individual headaches, frequency, quality of pain or discomfort, precipitating or aggravating factors (e.g. reading) and whether relieved by analgesics. With practice, these details take little time to elicit: nowhere in medicine is the history more important than in headache, partly because physical signs are often absent. Occasionally an early presbyope or hypermetrope will present with frontal headache after 15 minutes of reading, relieved by stopping reading but recurring when reading is resumed.

Of course, severe pain in the eye will be accompanied by periorbital or forehead pain (e.g. in acute closed-angle glaucoma and corneal ulceration), but the patient will seldom mention it.

Inappropriate Referrals

The ophthalmologist sometimes receives inappropriate referrals.

Trigeminal neuralgia is one. Elderly patients have very sudden attacks *lasting literally a second or two* of pain in and behind one eye. Sometimes a precipitating factor can be identified, e.g. exposure to cold or even mere touch. At first, frequency is once in a few weeks but it increases gradually until attacks occur daily or even more often. The eye itself is white and has good acuity which, with the very short duration of the episodes of pain, excludes closed-angle glaucoma. When the maxillary division of the trigeminal (Vth) nerve is affected, the otolaryngology department may receive the patient; the dentist may well be involved if the mandibular division is affected.

Frontal sinusitis can also be mistaken for acute closed-angle glaucoma. Right or left low frontal pain usually starts at a particular time, e.g. mid-morning, with remarkable regularity for a week or so before it drives the patient to his doctor. The pain builds up over an hour or so to reach a plateau, presumably because the ostium is blocked by muco-pus when the patient is erect. Recumbency or sleep, following analgesics, often relieves the pain, presumably because free drainage from the sinus is re-established, the thick muco-pus having gravitated away from the exit. Pressure by the examiner's thumb gently but firmly upwards under the medial end of the eyebrow will usually elicit tenderness.

Migraine may propel the patient to the eye clinic even if he or she has no 'fortification spectrum' or other visual aura: a jagged shimmering arc in one homonymous half-field or quadrant may appear and last a few minutes before the headache starts. Age is important: onset is very commonly in the late 'teens, very seldom after the mid-twenties. The patient usually makes the diagnosis himself because the inheritance is dominant, but with variable penetrance and expressivity. The distribution is often frontal, usually unilateral, involving the area of the eye. Although unilateral in any attack, it is *very* rare for the same side *always* to be affected and *never* the other side (in contrast to cluster headaches). Nausea and even vomiting often accompany the headache, which lasts a few hours. Effective treatment offers a therapeutic test that can also be applied to other less common 'vascular' neuralgias, e.g. cluster headaches. Spectacles in our experience do not cure migraine.

All clinicians tend to develop two neuroses — justifiably — when presented with a 'headache' patient: *intracranial aneurysm and intracranial tumour*. Both of these are beyond the scope of this book. Again the history is important. Catastrophic suddenness and great severity, with diplopia (pressure on IIIrd, IVth, Vth or VIth are frequent) are almost diagnostic of the former. Neck stiffness and more diffuse headache suggest a leak of blood into the subarachnoid space. Intracranial tumour, with many exceptions, tends to have a short history of morning frontal headache increasing quickly in severity and duration over a period of 6–8–10 weeks; vomiting and papilloedema (often unilateral at first) appear relatively late to complete the typical triad.

Chapter 10

Diabetes and the Eye

Diabetic eye disease is possibly the most important single subject within ophthalmic practice for two reasons: it is the commonest cause of blindness in the working population (aged 20 – 60 years), and most cases are preventable or treatable. In the absence of treatment, diabetic eye disease may cause irreversible ocular damage, and it is therefore essential for the non-specialist to understand the mechanisms by which diabetes mellitus affects vision, ·and the simple principles of management. Ocular complications occur in patients with both insulin-dependent (IDDM) and non-insulin-dependent diabetes mellitus (NIDDM), but diabetic eye disease usually presents earlier in the former. The prevalence of ocular complications directly attributable to diabetes has not been accurately defined, although evidence of retinopathy in various stages has been demonstrated in at least 80% of insulin-dependent diabetics within 20 years of diagnosis.

Diabetes mellitus has been associated with a myriad of ocular complications, including iritis, iridopathy of the iris muscles, autonomic neuropathy of the iris causing abnormal pupil reactions, occlusion of the retinal veins, optic neuritis and papillitis, and extraocular muscle palsies secondary to neuropathy of the IIIrd, IVth and VIth cranial nerves. *However, the main causes of impaired vision attributable to diabetes are retinopathy, cataracts and glaucoma.*

Retinopathy

Retinopathy in diabetes is part of a generalized microvascular disease that also affects the kidneys (nephropathy) and the peripheral nerves (neuropathy). Regular detailed ophthalmoscopic examination of the retina is essential in diabetic patients. Further information on retinal integrity may be obtained from fluorescein angiography, in which a small dose of fluorescein is injected into a peripheral arm vein, and photographs are taken of the retina at one-second intervals to demonstrate abnormalities in retinal blood flow and leakage of fluorescein from damaged areas of the retina. See Fig. 10.1.

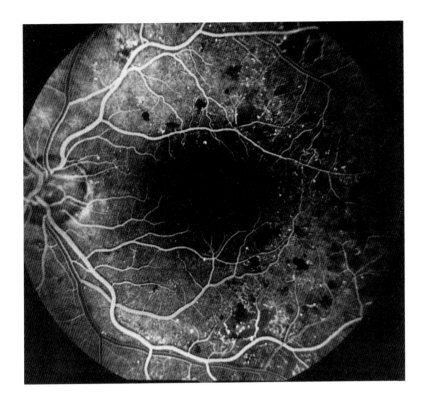

Fig. 10.1. A 'fluorescein fundus photograph'. After an IV injection of fluorescein has been given, at one-second intervals a series of photographs of the fundus is taken, using an input of blue light (420–490 mm) through an 'exciting' filter to activate this dye. All emitted light is filtered out except for the yellow-green at 510–530 mm by a 'barrier' filter so that a high contrast black and white photograph is obtained. The *normal* retinal blood vessels do not allow leakage of the dye because it has rapidly combined with the plentiful albumin.

This angiogram of 'background diabetic retinopathy' shows microaneurysms and areas of capillary closure. The arterioles are completely filled (white) with dye-containing blood that is just starting to reach the venules in white ribbons.

Diabetic retinopathy is classified into the following major categories: (a) background retinopathy, (b) maculopathy, (c) proliferative retinopathy. Patients found to have (b) and (c), including pre-proliferative signs described below, should be referred urgently to an ophthalmologist: a non-ophthalmologist may monitor (a) but exudates between the supero-temporal and infero-temporal branches of the central retinal artery warrant urgent specialist referral, because they threaten the macula. Subnormal visual acuity (VA) with spectacles, if worn, is another indication for referral unless there is some other explanation, e.g. strabismic amblyopia.

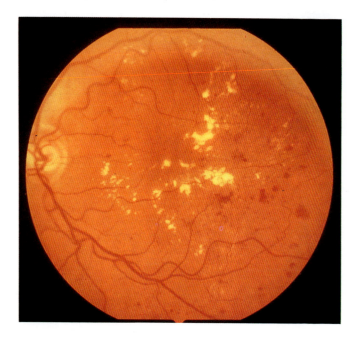

Fig. 10.2. Severe 'background diabetic retinopathy' with microaneurysms, dot haemorrhages and extensive hard exudates in the macular area, hence very reduced visual acuity. See Fig. 10.1 for a fluorescein fundus photograph of an earlier stage.

Background Diabetic Retinopathy

Pathological changes in the diabetic retina follow microvascular leakage, which leads to intraretinal haemorrhage and oedema (Fig. 10.2). The characteristic features of background retinopathy are the following.

Microaneurysms
These are discrete, localized saccular distensions of the weakened capillary walls, presenting as small, circular red 'dots' in the retina. Microaneurysms tend to be the first ophthalmoscopically-detectable sign of diabetic retinopathy. They are particularly well demonstrated by fluorescein angiography (Fig. 10.1).

Intraretinal Haemorrhages

Impairment of the blood–retina barrier, i.e. the tight junctions between the endothelial cells of the retinal blood vessels, causes patchy leakage of the vascular contents into the retina. The appearance of the haemorrhage is dependent upon its position within the retina: haemorrhages deep within the retina are tightly enclosed by the surrounding retinal structures, and therefore appear as small circular 'dot' haemorrhages, whilst superficial haemorrhages in the nerve fibre layer follow the course of the nerve fibres and appear as 'flame-shaped' haemorrhages, which characteristically have a 'feathery' edge. (Fig. 10.2).

Hard Exudates

Leakage from retinal vessels — especially microaneurysms — also leads to the accumulation of intraretinal oedema. Discrete, well-defined, white-yellow 'hard exudates', consisting of lipids and lipoproteins, are deposited at the periphery of the localized areas of retinal oedema (Fig. 10.2).

Unless and until the haemorrhages and exudates involve the fovea, there is usually no subjective effect on visual acuity. Treatment of this condition is essentially preventive, with stable maintenance of diabetic control and careful treatment of complications associated with diabetes, e.g. hypertension. There is no ocular treatment for background diabetic retinopathy.

Maculopathy

'Diabetic maculopathy' is applied when background diabetic retinopathy affects the macular area. It is the commonest cause of visual impairment in diabetes, and is particularly associated with the non-insulin-dependent form of the disease. It is subdivided into the following categories.

- *Focal maculopathy*, where there is a specific area of microvascular leakage. This presents clinically as hard exudate formation, usually in a circular pattern ('circinate retinopathy') with the leaking point in the centre of the ring of exudate. Providing the fovea is not involved, there may be no subjective loss of vision. Treatment consists of accurate localization of the leaking point by fluorescein angiography, followed by application of laser treatment to destroy the leaking vessel to prevent further leakage.
- *Oedematous maculopathy* describes a condition of diffuse leakage from macular capillaries, resulting in the accumulation of oedema at the

macula. Attempts to treat this condition by laser photocoagulation have not proved particularly successful, although some cases are improved by application of a 'grid' of laser burns over the macula (avoiding the fovea).

● *Ischaemic maculopathy* is due to capillary non-perfusion within the macula. There are no clinical diagnostic features, and it can be definitively diagnosed only by fluorescein angiography. Again there is no effective treatment for this form of maculopathy.

Proliferative Retinopathy

Proliferative retinopathy refers to the development of new vessels in the retina in response to significant retinal ischaemia, and is the most serious complication of diabetes. A vasoproliferative polypeptide derived from ischaemic retina is the stimulus to neovascularization. It affects less than 5% of the diabetic population, *but it has a poor visual prognosis if treatment is not started at an early stage in the disease process.*

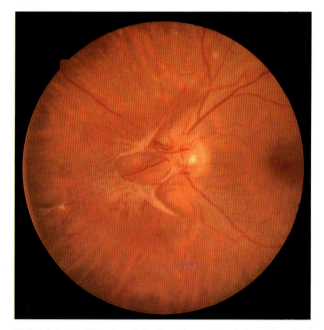

Fig. 10.3. Proliferative diabetic retinopathy. A large frond of new blood vessels with fibrous tissue has grown out from the optic disc into the vitreous in response to a vasculogenic polypeptide that has diffused out from ischaemic areas of retina. Fortunately, the macula (dark disc at the edge of the picture) is not obscured.

This condition may be preceded by *pre-proliferative retinopathy*, of which the most characteristic feature is 'cottonwool spots'. These are white, fluffy lesions usually situated at the posterior pole of the eye near the optic disc, and represent a failure of normal axoplasmic transport within the nerve fibres as a result of ischaemia. A collection of swollen axons constitutes a cottonwool spot. Although there is no treatment for this pre-proliferative retinopathy, these patients should be regularly examined at short intervals as a proportion of them will progress to the development of overt retinal neovascularization.

Proliferative retinopathy is subdivided according to the position of the new vessels in the retina into neovascularization of the optic disc and neovascularization in the retinal periphery. Disc neovascularization has the worse prognosis, and serious loss of vision will develop within 2 years in at least 40% of untreated diabetic patients with this condition. Treatment consists of pan-retinal photocoagulation using a laser, in which the whole of the retina apart from the macula is obliterated by confluent laser burns. This therapy destroys the ischaemic retina, and so removes the stimulus to the proliferation of new blood vessels; the vessels usually regress. Surprisingly, the loss of this large area of the retina causes less impairment of vision than one would anticipate, and the commonest subsequent visual problems are constriction of the peripheral visual field and impairment of night vision. Most importantly, the central visual acuity is preserved, and therefore most patients can enjoy a reasonably normal lifestyle.

Peripheral neovascularization, the development of new vessels from retinal veins, is not as serious as new vessels at the optic disc. Pan-retinal photocoagulation is also required in most cases, and the prognosis for maintenance of moderate visual acuity is generally very good.

Unlike the normal retinal vasculature, the new blood vessels are extremely fragile. Unless neovascularization is treated in the early stages of the disease process, these vessels have a tendency to leak and rupture, producing haemorrhage into the vitreous.

Loss of vision occurs in untreated diabetic patients from the following.

- Vitreous haemorrhage.
- Tractional retinal detachment, caused by contraction of fibrovascular membranes (often initiated by vitreous haemorrhage) on the retina, which literally pull the neurosensory retina from its normal anatomical location. Tears in the retina are sometimes a consequence of a pathological process, rather than the predisposing cause (as in rhegmatogenous, that is hole-produced, retinal detachment: p.115).

- Neovascular glaucoma, which is a painful form of glaucoma characterized by new vessels on the iris. The fibrovascular membrane also occludes the trabecular meshwork. This is particularly refractory to treatment, and may require enucleation. See p. 78.

Although the severe complications of proliferative diabetic retinopathy are amenable to treatment with recent developments in intraocular surgery (vitrectomy), if the macula is involved the prognosis for visual acuity remains poor and the best result that may be obtained is maintenance of 'navigating vision' for the patient. Vitrectomy may be indicated when vascularized fibrous tissue has invaded the vitreous cavity or has grown over the surface of the retina, and would not respond to laser treatment. The surgeon can excise these membranes, using ophthalmoscopes and the operation microscope; his microsurgical instruments gain access usually through the sclera and 'pars plana' of the retina, i.e. in the far periphery of the fundus, anterior to the peripheral edge of the retina proper but behind the iris–lens diaphragm. It is therefore essential to emphasize that most ocular complications of diabetes may be prevented by careful diabetic control, regular ocular examination, and early intervention, especially with laser treatment. Accordingly, diabetic eye disease should be regarded as a preventable form of blindness in the majority of patients.

Cataracts

Although lens opacification (cataract) has been described virtually as an overnight phenomenon in poorly controlled diabetics, the usual effect of diabetes on the lens is to accelerate 'senile' cataract, causing lens opacification to occur at a relatively younger age. The commonest types of cataract associated with diabetes are nuclear lens opacification, in the centre of the lens, and posterior subcapsular lens opacity, in the posterior aspect of the lens. Cataract formation and treatment are described in Chapter 8.

Glaucoma

Glaucoma, particularly open-angle glaucoma, is a silent, insidious form of progressive blindness that may only become symptomatic in the late stages of the disease process (see Chapter 5). Diabetes mellitus is associated with both open-angle and closed-angle glaucoma, as well as 'neovascular' (one kind of 'secondary') glaucoma described above and also on p. 78.

Chapter 11

TRAUMA

General Comments

The eyeball is a very exposed and very delicate part of the central nervous system, extremely vulnerable to injuries. Before we consider these systematically, some general comments are worth making, often applicable to injuries in general.

Most injuries are fortunately trivial though frequent. More serious injuries are so disabling, painful and 'expensive' in patients' and doctors' time and other scarce resources, that *preventive measures* of every sort would pay dividends. That raises the question of risk-taking, e.g. boxing and squash rackets.

The small proportion of one-eyed individuals in the population (e.g. those with strabismic amblyopia) should obviously take even fewer risks than the average two-eyed person.

As much detailed history as possible should be obtained, especially to assess sources of contamination of wounds: for example, agricultural injuries alert us to possible fungus infection. A child's history — if any is available — may be understandably distorted to protect his siblings or friends.

Particularly when dealing with unconscious patients, be aware of the potentially disastrous effects of corneal exposure. Corneal drying occurs within minutes, corneal ulceration within a day or so, panophthalmitis and blindness after 2–3 days. This can be prevented simply by taping the eyelids closed. If this is impossible or impractical, apply an antibiotic oculentum every 3–4 hours.

The state of the pupils is an important sign in the management of head injury and coma, so do NOT use mydriatics to see the fundus in such patients. See p. 129.

Facial injuries and fractures, often with swollen rigid eyelids, impose three responsibilities on the doctor, especially if the patient is or has been unconscious: to ensure that the eyeball has normal visual acuity and is intact (lid retractors inserted under topical anaesthesia, with extreme care to avoid damaging the cornea, may well be essential); to exclude *blow-out fracture* of the floor of the orbit (palpate carefully for tenderness, crepitus and subcutaneous emphysema along the lower orbital margin); and to check other systems, from ribs and spleen to ankles, for other injuries. In suspected orbital blow-out fracture, a few days' delay is permissible before a forced duction test under topical anaesthesia is done to confirm tethering of the inferior rectus muscle in the fracture; with plain forceps grasp the conjunctiva just below the cornea and try to rotate the eyeball upwards: failure indicates blow-out fracture. On radiography an opaque maxillary sinus (due to blood) is very suspicious, or soft orbital tissue prolapsed into the sinus may be visible. Note that a radiograph may miss a fracture in the complex facial bones.

Fortunately most injuries are unilateral. For that reason, in later life trauma should be suspected as the original cause if a patient presents with unilateral open-angle glaucoma or unilateral cataract, etc.

Depending on the cause of the injury and the patient's immunological status in relation to tetanus, a 'booster' dose of toxoid may be indicated; if specific (passive) immunoglobulin is required, a subsequent course of active immunization should be given.

Eyelids

An apparently innocent minor lacerated wound, especially of the upper lid, may occasionally mislead the *general* casualty officer into missing a perforating wound of the underlying eyeball: simply lifting the upper lid and inspecting the eyeball closely with a good light will usually suffice to avoid that mistake. Similarly, the *ophthalmic* casualty officer should think of a *deep* injury, especially in a child: a sharp stick or metal spike may pierce the eyelid, enter the orbit, then penetrate the orbital plate of the frontal bone to injure a frontal lobe and start meningitis or brain abscess with or without a retained intracranial foreign body.

Even quite severe lacerated wounds of the eyelids are usually easily sutured and heal well with little risk of secondary infection because of the good blood supply. Cosmetically the results are usually very good. Wounds at the nasal end of the lower lid may tear the lower canaliculus (which is difficult to repair), and carry the risk of permanent epiphora: the upper canaliculus is much less important. The risk of distortion of the eyelashes should be minimized at operation because they may rub on the cornea or conjunctiva and later require regular epilation, electrolysis or cryotherapy.

Foreign Bodies

Conjunctival Foreign Bodies

For these, which are very common, the history is diagnostic: pain in one eye after grit was blown in by a gust of wind. With a good light and reading spectacles if worn to allow *close* inspection, retract the lower lid gently and the small foreign body will usually be seen in the lower fornix and easily removed with a sterile swab stick or cotton bud. The next easiest site to inspect is the *whole* cornea — make sure to lift the upper lid. Then suspect a subtarsal foreign body, i.e. one that is underneath the upper lid so that blinking exacerbates the pain. Eversion of the upper lid is an apparently simple technique which requires practice and attention to detail: see Fig. 11.1. Students should use each other as patients. After removal of the foreign body, an antibiotic oculentum should be prescribed three times daily for 2–3 days and the patient should be warned to return if the discomfort has not gone in 12–24 hours.

Corneal Foreign Bodies

These are common but must be treated very carefully mainly because infection can occasionally convert a trivial injury to a disaster. See Fig. 6.2. The history is usually the same as in conjunctival foreign bodies above, but a buff or a lathe or similar machine at work may be the source (see also intraocular foreign body below). Such an occupational foreign body will have been red-hot when given off, and therefore sterile. Removal is usually easy by means of a sterile cotton bud — with

---

Fig. 11.1 (overleaf). Technique of eversion of the left upper lid and removal of subtarsal foreign body. Students should practise on each other. (a) The patient lies on a couch with one thin pillow. The operator, *of course*, washes his hands thoroughly and scrubs his nails, then stands behind the top of the patient's head. The patient is asked to look downwards towards her feet. (b) The free end of a sterile swabstick in the operator's right hand is placed 5–6 mm above the lash margin, i.e. at the upper border of the upper tarsal plate, to act as a fulcrum round which the left thumb and index finger rotate the upper lid. The operator's left thumb pulls the skin of the upper lid laterally and slightly upwards to disengage the lid margin from the eyeball. (Most clinicians merely grasp the eyelashes.) (c) The left index finger is used to push the margin of the lower lid up underneath the edge of the upper lid. Moderate pressure by the left thumb contributes to the fulcrum being applied by the swabstick, both of which push the upper margin of the upper lid's tarsal plate downwards until (d) the upper lid turns inside out. (e) The other end of the swabstick (still sterile, not having been touched) is then used to remove any subtarsal foreign body. (f) Finally, the margin of the lower lid is used as a fixed point on to which the edge of the everted upper tarsal plate is pressed so that the upper lid flips back into its normal position.

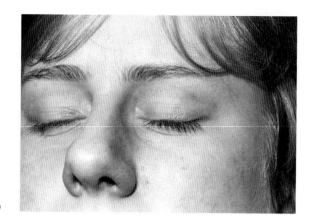

11.1 (a)

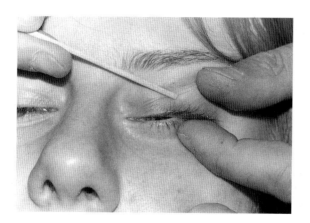

11.1 (b)

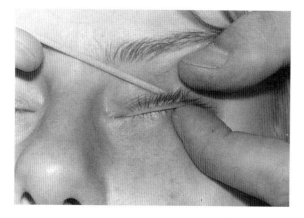

11.1 (c)

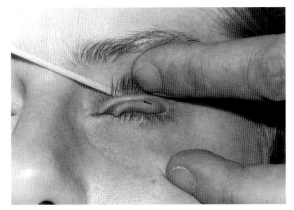

11.1 (d)

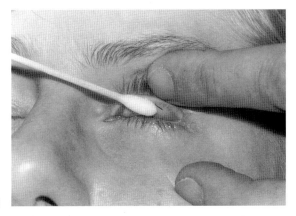

11.1 (e)

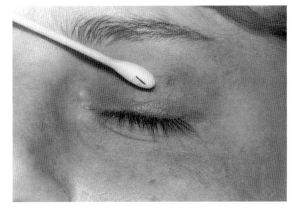

11.1 (f)

a good light shone obliquely on the eye to avoid dazzling the patient; several instillations of a topical anaesthetic with 2–3 minutes of closed eyelids should precede the operation. Failure to dislodge the foreign body indicates immediate referral, preferably to a specialist eye unit where magnification and good lighting are available: a sterile disposable needle on a small sterile disposable syringe will prick it out. An antibiotic oculentum 2–3 times daily and a sterile pad taped over the eye to keep the eyelids closed for a day or so are usually prescribed. The patient should be seen at least once about 24–36 hours later to check for signs of early corneal ulceration, which is a slough developing at the site of damage to the cornea, accompanied by an increasingly painful eye with conjunctival hyperaemia, especially circumcorneal (see Fig. 6.2).

Intraocular Foreign Bodies
These are important because even small ones can be very destructive and are easily missed. You should suspect these especially in a patient who has been operating a lathe or using a hammer and chisel. The patient may report only a transient feeling of a foreign body entering the eye. Be particularly careful if no conjunctival or corneal foreign body is found. The visual acuity may be normal, but may already be reduced by early cataract resulting from perforation of the lens capsule. Such a patient should be sent immediately to ophthalmic A&E where the high magnification and intense illumination of the slit-lamp microscope may allow the ophthalmologist to see a tiny oblique perforating wound of cornea, before the patient goes for radiography. Larger intraocular foreign bodies produce more obvious perforating corneal or scleral wounds, distortion of the pupil or frank prolapse of iris, obvious cataract and very reduced visual acuity. Early diagnosis is essential, especially for unsterile foreign bodies which usually come from a hammer or chisel rather than from the material being worked: a metal fragment from a lathe is red hot at source and therefore sterile. Removal under general anaesthesia is usually easily possible with a magnet, followed over a period of months or years by cataract extraction and sometimes repair of retinal detachment. Prognosis for ultimate vision in all such cases should be guarded.

Cornea

Corneal Ulceration
Corneal ulceration is serious and requires immediate specialist treatment because eventual corneal opacification and distortion must be

minimized and because the infection (staphylococci, pneumococci and *Pseudomonas pyocyaneus* are the common organisms) may well quickly move inside the eyeball. See Fig. 6.2. (Trauma seldom introduces a virus, but fungi are a risk especially from agricultural injuries, and produce a chronic inflammation that is difficult to treat.) A frankly purulent discharge and spreading corneal opacification from the ulcer covered by a slough are typical: the eye is painful and the conjunctiva angrily hyperaemic. A swab and smear, and culture for sensitivities, should be taken before intensive local and systemic broad-spectrum antibiotics are given. Inflammatory products diffuse through the cornea and aqueous humour to elicit an inflammatory response from the iris: there are many white cells in the exudate that can be seen as glinting particles in the anterior chamber with the slit-lamp microscope. When they gravitate and aggregate, the observer's naked eye can see the yellowish deposit with a fluid level at the bottom of the anterior chamber — an hypopyon: note that organisms need not enter the eyeball itself to produce this appearance, i.e. septic endophthalmitis need not quite be diagnosed at that stage. See Fig. 6.2. If and when infection does spread deeply into the eyeball, intraocular antibiotics and/or vitrectomy are drastic methods that may save some sight, but evisceration may be necessary to prevent septicaemia and meningitis. In evisceration, all the intraocular contents are scraped out after excision of the cornea. In the actively infected stage, enucleation — removal of the whole eyeball — is contraindicated because of the risk of meningitis when the optic nerve is cut.

In the longer term, a healed corneal ulcer or keratitis usually reduces visual acuity considerably, and may produce an unsightly scar. Fortunately, the other eye is usually normal so that corneal grafting may not be required; it has a rather poor prognosis anyway because the injured cornea is usually vascularized, which predisposes to graft rejection (see pp. 121 and 122).

Corneal Abrasion
Corneal abrasion is also common and usually heals within a few days, with one longer-term occasional complication. See Fig. 11.2. A glancing sweep with a newspaper or a child's finger denudes some of the cornea of epithelium. There is great pain and watering. To confirm the diagnosis (using single-dose sterile formulations to prevent cross-infections),

- instil a topical anaesthetic to make the patient comfortable;
- instil fluorescein eye drops;
- instil a few saline eye drops to wash out excess fluorescein: the damaged area of cornea retains the stain;

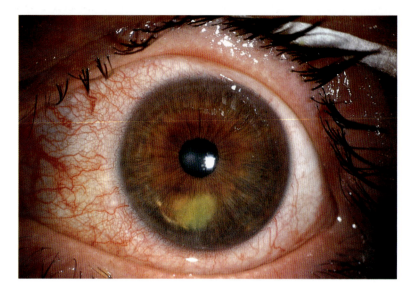

Fig. 11.2. Corneal abrasion stained with fluorescein eye drops, the excess 'washed off' with two or three drops of saline eye drops. Note the diffuse conjunctival hyperaemia.

- inspect the cornea with a bright light from a pen-torch, ophthalmoscope, etc. and observe the abraded area stained bright green.

An antibiotic oculentum daily with a sterile eye pad taped to the face and replaced daily holds the eyelid shut and helps to prevent infection that would convert a simple abrasion into a serious ulcer.

Occasionally, for unknown reasons, a few weeks or even months after healing of a simple corneal abrasion, the epithelium covering the healed area is lifted up like a trap-door, usually when the eyelids are opened on waking in the morning. The exact symptoms of the original abrasion recur, but only for a few hours, which suggests that the trap-door of epithelium quickly falls back into place. Every few weeks or days, *'recurrent corneal abrasion'* will produce its unpleasant symptoms. An antibiotic oculentum at night for 4–6 weeks as a lubricant will usually suffice, but the more drastic cauterization of the affected area, if it can be identified, may be necessary to cause a mild inflammation that allows the epithelium to obtain a permanent grip on its bed.

Contact lenses are a common cause of corneal abrasions. Most heal quickly, but all contact lens wearers must have usable glasses available so that the contact lenses can be removed *from both eyes* as soon as any new discomfort appears. Opportunisitic colonization by pathogens including pyogens and fungi may cause corneal ulceration, especially in users of soft or extended-wear contact lenses (see p. 31).

Chemical Burns
Alkalis, for example lime on a building site, are the most serious and common. Immediate — first-aid — irrigation of the conjunctival sac(s) with plenty of clear water should be done if possible, but blepharospasm may be difficult to overcome: a topical anaesthetic would help, at least in mild cases. Emergency treatment in hospital employs saline irrigation and picks off pieces of alkali from the conjunctival sac: double eversion of the upper lid is required to clean out the recesses of the upper fornix. Anaesthesia with cocaine eye drops is usually effective. Unfortunately, alkali penetrates the cornea quickly and provokes keratitis and fibrosis; heavy neovascularization from the limbus indicates a poor prognosis for corneal grafting in the long term — the lymphatics that accompany the blood vessels explain the frequent host-graft reaction. See p. 121. A chronic progressive ulceration may ensue in spite of efficient cleansing because the alkali removes the inhibitor of collagenase (released from injured cells), which can then digest collagen, the main constituent of cornea: cysteine eye drops may halt the process. In contrast, acids tend to be bound by tissue protein, which limits penetration, so that irrigation to remove the excess residual acid usually suffices.

Eyeball Concussion
This is a common injury especially in children at play with balls. A traumatic hyphaema (blood in the anterior chamber) is the equivalent of a bruise. The extravasion of blood from the iris may be enough to accumulate at 6 o'clock in the anterior chamber, with a fluid level. See Fig. 11.3. A small hyphaema will absorb untreated in a few days, with rest to minimize the risk of the much more serious and larger — often total — 'secondary hyphaema'. A larger hyphaema, like a 'secondary', carries a strong risk of raised intraocular pressure because the outflow of aqueous humour is obstructed. 'Secondary glaucoma', in turn, adds to the risk of 'blood staining of the cornea'. To prevent that, reduction of intraocular pressure (by acetazolamide orally and β-blocking eye drops) and surgical irrigation of the anterior chamber may be indicated, but further recurrences of the bleeding may well occur. In the long term, damage to the trabecular meshwork by mere concussion, or by more direct damage by hyphaema, may produce a chronic glaucoma very like open-angle glaucoma, but fortunately unilateral.

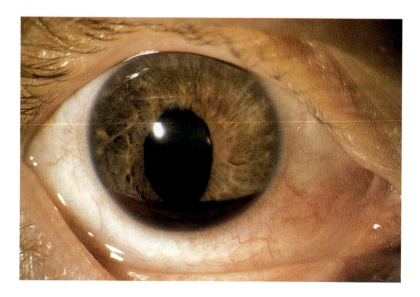

Fig. 11.3. Concussion hyphaema. A blow from a fast-moving squash ball has caused extravasation of blood from fragile iris vessels (or from a cleft in the ciliary body). The red cells have gravitated downwards. Note also the traumatic mydriasis (= dilatation of pupil) inferiorly, and the distortion of iris architecture (whorls) at 12 o'clock.

Macular oedema and choroidal tears (sometimes with intravitreous haemorrhage) are contre-coup lesions, like those in head injury.

Other long-term risks are (unilateral) cataract, with or without subluxation or complete dislocation of the lens, and traumatic retinal detachment.

Penetrating Injury
Sharp objects such as knives, or severe injuries with blunt objects may cause perforation or rupture of the eyeball. Its anterior segment is usually affected so that careful close inspection with a good light will usually reveal a lacerated wound of the cornea, often with a distorted pupil indicating a prolapsed iris which itself may be less obvious. The lens may become opaque quickly if its capsule is widely ruptured. Vitreous, like clear egg-white, spilling out from the wound indicates that the injury has extended behind the lens and its suspensory ligament. The history will usually indicate whether a retained intraocular foreign body may also be present. Of course, management demands emergency referral to an ophthalmic surgeon, but in the meantime avoid pressure on the eyeball or eyelids that might push out intraocular contents.

The first priority in treatment is to excise under general anaesthesia prolapsed intraocular contents, especially iris, and suture the wound of the corneo-scleral envelope. The damaged cataractous lens is also removed at the same time or later. Systemic and local antibiotics will reduce the risk of infection. In the longer term, corneal grafting may be indicated, but if the fellow eye is normal a more conservative approach is often adopted, especially because the long-term prognosis for useful vision is not good. Glaucoma and retinal detachment may be (late) complications.

Sympathetic Ophthalmitis
This is a fascinating disease. Starting 9 days or more after a *perforating* injury in one eye (peak interval about 3 months), a very small proportion of patients will develop a chronic inflammation of the iris, ciliary body and choroid (pan-uveitis) *in both eyes*. The risk is around 1:10000 and we cannot predict who will suffer.

The pathogenesis is not known exactly, but it seems likely that a perforating injury allows intraocular antigen(s), especially of uveal origin, to obtain access to lymphatics hitherto denied to them because there are no intraocular lymph vessels (just as there are no intracranial lymphatics). That unusual route is a factor in their being able to excite an autoimmune delayed (T cell) hypersensitivity response. These T cells attack all uveal tissue in *both* eyes. Surprisingly, there is no similar encephalitis following open head injury.

The tragic result is often blindness over a period of weeks, months or years, delayed by steroids and other immunosuppressive drugs. Glaucoma and cataract often appear as the disease progresses. Histologically the appearances are diagnostic. The earliest clinical sign is white cells seen by the slit-lamp microscope in the anterior chamber of the injured *and* fellow eye. Ophthalmologists managing a perforating injury have a 'nine-day neurosis' because removal of the injured eye within nine days of the injury will protect completely against sympathetic ophthalmitis. The reason for this latent period is unknown. The authors prefer to enucleate a badly injured eye that has little chance of useful vision within that period rather than take even the small risk of sympathetic ophthalmitis. More difficult is the management of a less serious injury, but urgent and careful suturing of corneo-scleral perforations and elimination of incarcerated or prolapsed uveal tissue will minimize the risk. The commonest perforating injury is of course surgical, e.g. cataract extraction, but the risk of sympathetic ophthalmitis from a short surgical operation in which disturbed iris has been carefully re-positioned and the incision meticulously sutured is much less than from an irregular perforating accidental wound in which uveal tissue has been trapped for hours or days pending operation.

Enucleation

If the remaining eye has normal acuity and field, the loss of one eye produces surprisingly little visual disability: loss of some field on that side and loss of stereoscopic vision. The cosmetic handicap can be minimized by an artificial eye well matched to the normal one. The quite capacious socket, lined by conjunctiva (maximally conserved when the eyeball was removed) may allow the artificial eye to sink backwards unless specially designed. To provide support, at the operation for enucleation, a plastic ball may be implanted in the muscle cone to replace some of the bulk of the eyeball. A magnet may be incorporated to impart some movement in the artificial eye — its immobility being part of the cosmetic handicap. To reduce the risk of contracted socket in the long term, an artificial eye is best worn 24 hours a day but removed with very clean hands for twice-daily washing with low-scented toilet soap, then thorough rinsing with tap water. Most patients thus avoid infections, but some have episodes of conjunctivitis that should be treated promptly; a useful drug, with mainly antiseptic properties, is propamidine isethionate 0.1% (Brolene) as eye drops every one or two hours during the day, and oculentum at night. Ideally these drops should be generously instilled after the artifical eye has been removed and with the patient lying horizontally.

Chapter 12

THE EYELIDS

The eye and optic nerve — an extension of the central nervous system — are only moderately well protected by the bony orbital walls. A property of the sclera is protection of the choroid and retina, while the conjunctiva protects the anterior sclera. The cornea, however, is more vulnerable. The eyelids protect the eye anteriorly; blinking maintains the moist tear film covering the cornea, while closure of the eyelids protects the cornea and anterior segment of the eye against most common injuries. Corneal exposure for more than a few minutes is extremely dangerous — drying, ulceration and panophthalmitis can evolve in minutes, hours, and a day or so respectively (see p. 145).

Anatomy

The eyelids are thin folds of skin, with a central layer of fibrous tissue (the tarsal plates) that maintains the shape of the lids. The margin of the eyelid is anatomically bisected by the 'grey line', a thin grey line that defines the junction of skin (anteriorly) with conjunctiva (posteriorly). The eyelashes are situated anteriorly, and the ducts of modified sebaceous glands (Meibomian glands) emerge posteriorly. The levator palpebrae superioris muscle (innervated by the IIIrd cranial nerve) elevates the upper lid, and the lids are closed by the orbicularis oculi muscle (innervated by the VIIth cranial nerve).

Disorders of the Eyelids

Disorders of the eyelids may be classified as inflammation, malposition of the eyelashes, malposition of the eyelids and tumours of the eyelids.

Inflammation

Inflammation affecting the eyelids may primarily involve the skin, the eyelid margin, or the glands within the eyelid.

SKIN INFECTION

Herpetic infections are the most important involving the skin around the eyelids.

Herpes simplex infection may occur in either a primary form, or as a recurrent infection. Primary herpes simplex usually presents as crops of vesicles involving the lids and periorbital region. The eye may be involved with a conjunctivitis, but this is not the main feature of the disease. Treatment consists of separate application of antiviral ointments to the skin (unguentum) and eye (oculentum) for 2–3 weeks; a common ointment in current practice is acyclovir.

Following a primary infection (which may be subclinical), the virus remains dormant in the trigeminal ganglion, with the potential to reactivate, particularly in response to stress or debility. The virus then passes along the Vth nerve to the eye, causing dendritic ulcers on the cornea, which has a characteristic appearance. See also p. 85 and Fig. 6.1. These are effectively treated by an antiviral ointment applied 5 times per day for 10–14 days. *Steroids must never be prescribed for this condition or for an eye that might have this condition.* Topical steroids cause the ulcer to enlarge rapidly, covering a significant proportion of the cornea within a very short period (Fig. 6.1). This condition has a very poor prognosis, and is, of course, completely avoidable.

Herpes zoster (shingles) ophthalmicus is caused by the varicella-zoster virus. This is the chickenpox virus, which may remain latent in the trigeminal ganglion for many years, reactivation occasionally occurring during periods of stress or debility. The virus travels down the first division of the Vth cranial nerve to causes a painful vesicular rash only in the distribution of that part of the nerve. The eye itself is involved in 50% of cases, with conjunctivitis, corneal ulceration, iritis, and rarely optic neuritis.

Treatment aims to attack the virus locally and to prevent secondary infection by applying

- antiviral ointment (unguentum) to the skin lesions in the vesicular stage (corneal ulcers are not sensitive to antiviral agents in this condition);
- steroid eye drops and antibiotic eye drops 3–4 times during the day (with careful monitoring for steroid complications, e.g. progressing corneal ulceration or opacification and, if continued for more than 4–6 weeks, glaucoma);
- antibiotic eye ointment (oculentum) at night.

INFLAMMATION OF THE EYELID MARGIN

Blepharitis is inflammation of the margin of the eyelid, and is usually classified as staphylococcal blepharitis, seborrhoeic blepharitis or allergic blepharitis.

Staphylococcal Blepharitis
This is a chronic inflammation of the eyelashes, characterized by erythema of the lid margin and small scales or crusts at the base of the lashes. Treatment consists of

- regular cleansing of the eyelid margins using a cotton-tipped applicator dipped in a warm solution of weak baby shampoo;
- antibiotic ointment applied to the eyelid margin four times per day for 10 days.

Seborrhoeic Blepharitis
Excessive secretion of lipids by the Meibomian glands is associated with inflammation of the lid margin and greasy scales at the lash roots. This often occurs with seborrhoeic dermatitis of the scalp. Treatment is similar to that of staphylococcal blepharitis (above), with cleansing of the lids and antibiotic ointment, but a course of systemic tetracycline is also prescribed to counteract the bacteria that are assumed to break down the lipids at the lid margin into the irritating fatty acids that precipitate the blepharitis.

Allergic Blepharitis
This is caused by chemical irritation, usually from cosmetics. Treatment is effected by avoidance of the offending agent.

INFLAMMATION OF THE EYELID GLANDS

The glands of the eyelid margin are susceptible to infection, usually by *Staphylococcus aureus*. The most common conditions in this category are the following.

External hordeolum ('stye'), an infection of a lash follicle and the associated sebaceous gland. *This common small abscess 'points' typically in line with the base of the eyelashes.* The lesion usually resolves with a course of antibiotic ointment and application of warm compresses.

Internal hordeolum is an acute inflammation of a Meibomian gland. *This small abscess is centred several millimetres from the lid margin and usually 'points' on the conjunctival surface of the eyelid, but occasionally on the skin surface.* Treatment is similar to that of an external hordeolum, although surgical drainage may be necessary in a small proportion of cases.

Chalazion, or Meibomian cyst (Fig. 12.1) is a firm nodule within the eyelid, presumably a chronic inflammatory response to blockage in the duct of a Meibomian gland. This is a common problem, and is easily treated by surgical incision and curettage under local anaesthesia. Excision is not required because the wall of the lesion consists of granulation tissue (compare sebaceous cyst, which has an epithelial lining, requiring careful excision).

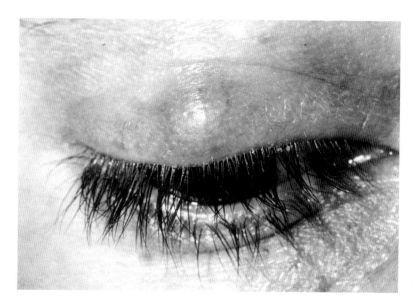

Fig. 12.1. Meibomian cyst (chalazion) of the upper eyelid.

Malposition of the Eyelashes

The eyelashes provide an additional line of protection for the eye, but are only effective in this function providing the lashes are directed away from the eye. If the eyelashes are distorted (trichiasis) and turn inwards towards the eye, they have an adverse effect, causing abrasion (and potentially ulceration) of the cornea. This may occur congenitally, but is commoner in the elderly, usually associated with scarring of the lid margin. See Fig. 15.4. Treatment consists of removal of the offending lashes, by epilation in the initial stages and by electrolysis or cryotherapy if recurrence is a major problem.

Malposition of the Eyelids

ENTROPION

An entropion is an inward rotation of the margin of the eyelid. (Fig. 12.2). The eyelashes abrade the cornea in this position, and therefore surgical correction is necessary. The most important cause of entropion of the lower eyelid is ageing, hence 'senile' or 'spastic' entropion with laxity of the lid tissues aggravated by spasm of the palpebral part of the orbicularis oculi muscle. A simple surgical procedure is required to correct the deformity, but the condition may recur.

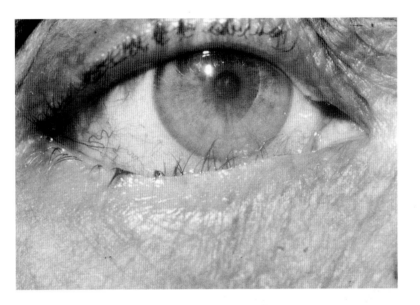

Fig. 12.2. 'Senile' entropion of the right lower lid. The eyelashes irritate the cornea and conjunctiva.

Scarring of the lid margin (cicatricial entropion) usually results from chemical burns (in Western countries) and trachoma (in the Third World; see Figs. 15.3 and 15.4) and may affect both upper and lower eyelids. Surgical correction is often required and is more extensive than for senile entropion.

ECTROPION

An ectropion is an outward rotation of the eyelid, margin (Fig. 12.3). This eyelid position prevents normal lid closure, which may lead to exposure of the cornea, while eversion of the lacrimal punctum causes watering of the eye, a common symptom. The causes of this condition are similar to those of entropion (ageing, with spasticity, and scarring of the lid margin), but to this must be added paralytic ectropion, due to paralysis of the facial nerve. Surgical correction is usually necessary to ensure adequate lid closure and corneal protection, especially at night, as well as cosmetic improvement; however, an antibiotic oculentum applied 3 – 4 times daily and liberally at night may suffice, at least temporarily.

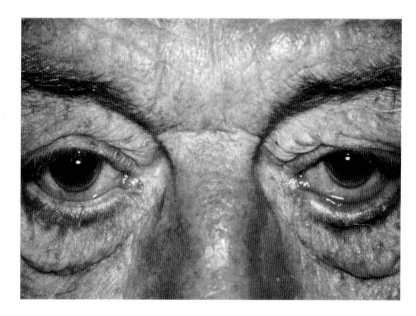

Fig. 12.3. Left senile ectropion of the lower lid with epiphora because the area of the lower lacrimal punctum is involved.

PTOSIS

Ptosis, or more accurately blepharoptosis, is applied to a drooping of the upper eyelid(s) (Fig. 12.4). Unlike entropion or ectropion, this form of eyelid malposition does not cause corneal exposure — quite the reverse.

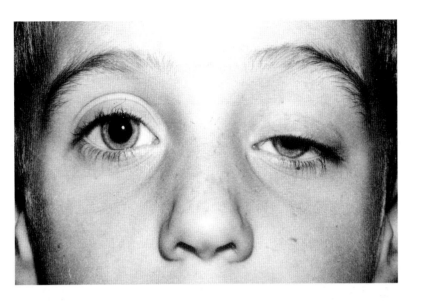

Fig. 12.4. Left congenital ptosis due to malfunction of the levator palpebrae superioris (LPS) muscle. Not surprisingly, the superior rectus muscle, which shares its embryological origin with the LPS, is sometimes also defective. In this case, the left eye showed poor elevation.

Although many cases are congenital, probably due to a defect in development of the levator palpebrae superioris muscle, most cases are acquired. The commonest causes of acquired ptosis are the result of

- 'mechanical' defects in the structures elevating the upper lid, e.g. senile weakness of the levator palpebrae superioris, or frank dehiscence of its aponeurosis;
- impairment of innervation to the muscles involved, e.g. IIIrd cranial nerve palsy or Horner's syndrome;
- muscular disease, e.g. myasthenia gravis.

Treatment is directed to the cause. In congenital cases and in mechanical disorders, surgical operation often corrects the defect, but neurogenic or myogenic causes require extensive investigation. As a general rule, myasthenia gravis should be considered and excluded in all cases of adult-onset ptosis prior to surgery. The usual operation consists of excision of a piece of the levator palpebrae superioris at its junction with the tarsal plate: in addition to the usual risks of operation, too much tissue may be excised, with danger of corneal exposure, or too little, with disappointment to all concerned.

EPICANTHUS

Epicanthus is the descriptive term for (congenital) vertical skin folds at the medial canthus (Fig. 12.5). This is not a true malposition of the eyelids; the appearance may result in a mistaken diagnosis of convergent squint. Most will spontaneously improve with normal development of the bridge of the nose.

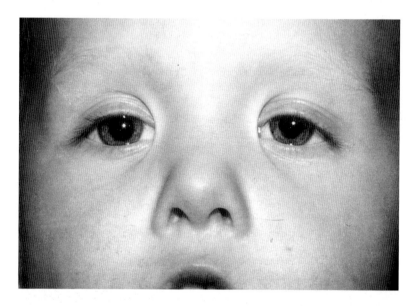

Fig. 12.5. Epicanthic folds. See also Fig 4.4. These usually disappear as the bridge of the nose develops.

Tumours of the Eyelids

Tumours of the eyelids are relatively common but seldom have an adverse prognosis. Benign tumours include solar and seborrhoeic keratosis, verrucae, and cutaneous horns, and are of little significance unless size merits excision. The commonest benign tumour is probably squamous papilloma, which presents as a slow-growing nodule within the skin. These may be excised as a minor procedure, although more extensive excision may be necessary in cases of late presentation.

Malignant tumours involving the skin adjacent to the eye are not uncommon in the elderly. These are usually basal cell carcinomas

(Fig. 12.6) but squamous cell carcinomas are not rare. Although the characteristic appearance of basal cell carcinoma, with an ulcerated crater surrounded by hyperkeratotic 'pearly' margin, is usually diagnostic, other forms of basal cell carcinoma are indistinguishable from squamous cell carcinoma. Treatment is similar in both cases, with adequate local excision, and has an excellent prognosis. There will be doubt about the diagnosis in many cases so that excision biopsy is often appropriate. Radiotherapy may be an alternative to surgery in basal cell carcinomas. As squamous cell carcinomas are not as sensitive to radiotherapy and — unlike basal cell carcinomas — have the potential to metastasize to regional lymph nodes, radiotherapy should be advocated only in cases where the diagnosis of basal cell carcinoma is confirmed, possibly by incisional biopsy.

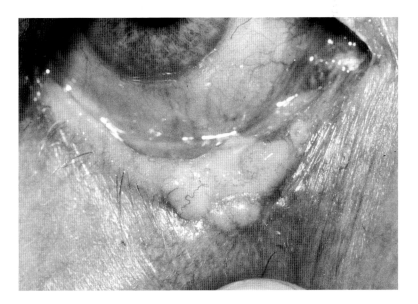

Fig. 12.6. Basal cell carcinoma of the right lower lid margin.

Chapter 13

THE ORBIT AND PROPTOSIS (EXOPHTHALMOS)

Orbital disease is uncommon, and conditions requiring surgery to the orbit are extremely rare; on average, only 5 patients per million of the population in the United Kingdom will require orbital surgery in a single year. However, it is important for the non-specialist to have the ability to identify those orbital conditions requiring urgent assessment. Fortunately, in this respect, orbital disease is amenable to relatively simple classification.

Applied Anatomy

The orbits are pyramidal bony cavities, base anteriorly, on the front of the skull, enclosed by bone on all sides except anteriorly. Any increase in the volume of the orbital contents can be accommodated only by forward protrusion of the eye (proptosis). There are sinuses on three sides, the maxillary sinus inferiorly, the ethmoidal sinuses medially, and the frontal sinus (and frontal lobe of the brain) superiorly. The lacrimal gland is situated anteriorly in the upper outer aspect of the orbit, and the eye is surrounded by the muscle cone and extraocular fat.

Symptoms and Aetiology of Orbital Disease

Any or all of proptosis (exophthalmos), diplopia, decrease in visual acuity, and discomfort or actual pain may be present.

AETIOLOGY OF ORBITAL DISEASE

(a) In children
- *Inflammatory.* Orbital infection (cellulitis) or oedema, produced by adjacent sinusitis.
- *Congenital* e.g. dermoid cysts and haemangiomas.
- *Neoplastic*, e.g. rhabdomyosarcoma, glioma, leukaemia.

(b) In adults
- Dysthyroid eye disease

- Vascular lesions. Orbital venous varices ('varicose veins of the orbit') and haemangiomas.
- Neoplasia; primary orbital neoplasms and metastatic deposits.
- Inflammatory disease usually from adjacent sinuses but occasionally 'orbital pseudo-tumour', a granulomatous inflammation of doubtful aetiology.
- Lacrimal gland lesions — inflammations or tumours (benign or malignant).

By far the commonest cause of proptosis, unilateral or bilateral, is dysthyroid eye disease, and is the only orbital condition of which the non-ophthalmologist need have detailed knowledge.

Diagnosis

The diagnostic approach to the differential diagnosis of orbital disease is relatively simple.

HISTORY

A short history of proptosis, particularly if associated with pain, is more suggestive of malignant or inflammatory disease; benign lesions tend to present with very slowly progressive proptosis and/or diplopia. Examination of old photographs is often useful in the identification of long-standing lesions.

EXAMINATION

Examination follows the standard routine of visual acuity, pupil reactions, ocular movements, visual fields, and ophthalmoscopy, all of which may be important in orbital disease depending on the site of the lesion. It is useful to stand behind the patient and look down towards the cornea over the frontal supra-orbital eminences; in unilateral proptosis, one cornea can be seen protruding beyond these eminences more than the other. To differentiate upper lid retraction from proptosis, inspect the patient's eyes from the front, with the patient gazing straight ahead: normally the edge of the lower lid crosses the corneo-scleral junction (limbus), whereas in proptosis the edge of the lower lid leaves a gap of white sclera visible below the limbus (Fig. 13.1).

Two further tests are necessary in the evaluation of orbital disease.

(1) Palpation of the region of the bony orbital margin, to detect anterior orbital lesions (especially lacrimal gland disorders at the upper outer rim of the orbit)

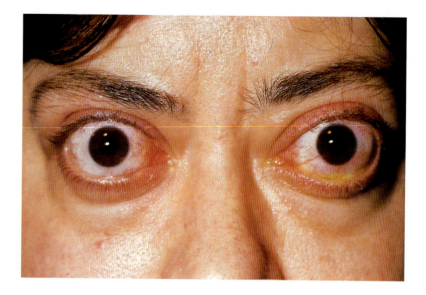

Fig. 13.1. Proptosis (exophthalmos) due to dysthyroid eye disease. The sclera can be seen between the lower lid margin and the limbus (corneo-scleral junction). Note that upper lid retraction is also present.

(2) Assessment of eyelid movements. These are of particular importance in the diagnosis of dysthyroid eye disease.

- *Lid retraction.* In the normal adult, the upper eyelid covers approximately 2 mm of the cornea; in dysthyroid eye disease, the upper lid is retracted, often allowing a small rim of white sclera to be visible above the cornea, thereby presenting a 'staring' appearance (Fig. 13.1).
- *Lid lag.* When the patient directs gaze downwards, there is a significant delay between the descent of the eye and the lesser and slower descent of the upper lid.

INVESTIGATIONS

Radiology
Radiography of the orbit from various angles permits differentiation of many orbital conditions. This information is supplemented by ultrasound of the orbit, computerized tomography, and magnetic resonance imaging. CT scanning is particularly useful in defining the exact site of the lesion in the orbit.

Haematology

Apart from blood counts and film, which are diagnostic of blood dyscrasias (particularly leukaemia), the most important haematological investigations are thyroid function tests: plasma concentrations of free T_4 and free T_3, and basal measurement of TSH by a sensitive assay.

Dysthyroid Eye Disease

Dysthyroid eye disease is the commonest cause of unilateral and bilateral proptosis, and must be considered in all cases of proptosis. It is a disease of middle age. The patients may be hyperthyroid, hypothyroid, or euthyroid at diagnosis, but patients have usually been hyperthyroid at some stage in the disease process. See Fig. 13.1.

Pathophysiology

Dysthyroid eye disease is an autoimmune disorder. Significant enlargement of the extraocular muscles and the orbital fat occurs as a result of infiltration of the tissues by lymphocytes, plasma cells, mast cells, and interstitial oedema. The bony orbit cannot accommodate this pathological increase in orbital contents, and therefore the eye is inevitably displaced anteriorly (proptosis).

Symptoms and Signs

Symptoms of hyperthyroidism are frequently present (sweating, tremor, weight loss, tachycardia), but dysthyroid eye disease may occur in patients with no other evidence of thyroid disease. Conjunctival vessels may be dilated, especially over the extraocular muscles. There is often asymmetrical retraction of the upper lids, giving the patient a staring appearance. Lid retraction and lid lag may be the only indicators of the disorder. Infiltration of the extraocular muscles causes restriction of eye movements, and diplopia is commonly the presenting symptom. The inferior rectus and medial rectus muscles are often the first to be involved, producing dioplopia in up-gaze (because the infiltrated inferior rectus cannot lengthen) and lateral gaze, but any muscle may be affected, and dysthyroid eye disease must be excluded (also myasthenia gravis) in any unusual case of diplopia. Proptosis is generally an obvious sign, and does not significantly affect vision in the majority of cases, but if the condition progresses, the increased volume of orbital contents may seriously impair vision by two mechanisms:

- Exposure of the cornea, as the eyelids are unable to cover the cornea in the grossly proptosed eye. *Corneal drying within minutes, ulceration within hours, and panophthalmitis within a day or so can quickly destroy the eye.*

- Compression of the optic nerve causing irreversible optic neuropathy.

Treatment

The manifestations of dysthyroid eye disease vary across a wide spectrum from mild to severe, and treatment is administered on an individual basis, according to the needs of the patient.

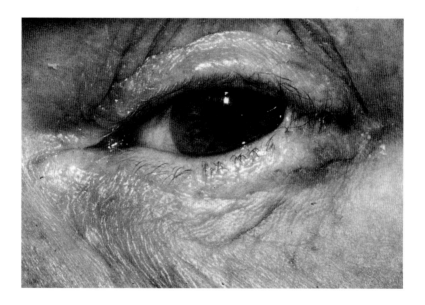

Fig. 13.2. Left eye. Lateral tarsorrhaphy to prevent corneal exposure in a case of left facial paralysis ('Bell's palsy'). The lateral ends of the upper and lower lid margins have been excised and sutured together. Occasionally a complete tarsorrhaphy has to be done, e.g. for chronic corneal ulcer or proptosis. When a tarsorrhaphy is opened, trichiasis is a risk.

- Artifical tears, for minimal conjunctival irritation. An oculentum at night is more protective during sleep.
- Surgical closure of the eyelids by tarsorrhaphy, to protect the cornea in more severe cases (Fig. 13.2). In tarsorrhaphy, the epithelium is excised from several millimetres of the upper and lower lid margins and the eyelids are sutured firmly together so that about seven days later the eyelids are joined together.

- Correction of diplopia, initially by prisms incorporated in spectacles, and finally by surgical squint operation(s).
- Treatment of corneal exposure, or optic neuropathy (an uncommon feature of dysthyroid eye disease) by decompression of the orbit, either medically (with high-dose steroids) or surgically.

Chapter 14

TEARS: THE DRY EYE AND THE WATERING EYE

The continuous production and drainage of tears is essential to the maintenance of a healthy eye. Tear flow subserves this function by four distinct mechanisms:

- continuous wetting of the cornea, thereby preventing the disastrous consequences of corneal desiccation;
- providing a smooth anterior corneal surface for optical clarity;
- protection against microorganisms by lysozymes and immuno-globulins;
- lubrication of the corneal surface, facilitating movements of the eyelids which also remove corneal debris and replace the tear film.

Obviously, disease may result from either tear deficiency (dry eye) or apparent tear excess (watering eye).

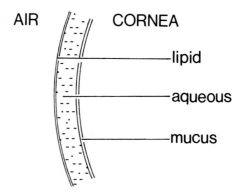

Fig. 14.1. Greatly magnified diagram of the normal tear-film. The mucin layer eliminates irregularities of the anterior surface of the corneal epithelium. The lipid layer reduces evaporation from the aqueous layer.

Normal Tear Film

Tears form a thin film over the anterior surface of the cornea that is frequently reconstituted by spontaneous blinking. The tear film has three layers (Fig. 14.1):

- A thin outer 'lipid layer' on the surface, produced by the Meibomian glands within the eyelids and released from the ducts on the eyelid margins. *This layer prevents evaporation of the underlying aqueous layer, thereby maintaining tear film stability.*
- A central 'aqueous layer' secreted by the lacrimal glands and comprising 90% of the depth of the tear film. There are two separate categories of lacrimal glands: the main lacrimal gland situated in the upper outer quadrant of the orbit, and the accessory lacrimal glands, which are multiple small glands situated in the conjunctival fornices. The accessory lacrimal glands have a very important role in the production of background basal secretion of tears essential to normal lubrication of the eye.
- A thin 'mucin layer' on the surface of the cornea. The mucin is produced by goblet cells in the conjunctiva and maintains adhesion between the aqueous layer of tears and the hydrophobic surface of the corneal epithelium.

The Dry Eye

If there is a deficiency of any component of the tear film, the cornea will become 'dry' during the intervals between blinking. The cornea is extremely sensitive, because of its extensive sensory innervation mediated by the Vth cranial nerve. The patient with a dry eye initially experiences grittiness and constant irritation, often associated with conjunctival inflammation (a non-infective conjunctivitis). These are the usual presenting symptoms of dry eyes, and are quite common in the elderly (see below). If this is not treated by tear replacement, erosions may appear on the corneal surface, possibly leading to corneal ulceration. Secondary infection with disastrous consequences is a potential complication. Very few patients progress further than the symptoms of grittiness in Western countries, but in Third World countries with a high prevalence of vitamin A deficiency, xerophthalmia (see p. 181) is a major cause of blindness.

The causes of dry eyes are classified according to the specific deficiencies in the components of the tear film.

(1) Diminished Production of the Aqueous Layer

Reduction in the aqueous component of tears is the most common cause of dry eyes, and occurs particularly in cases of rheumatoid arthritis (Sjögren syndrome). The diagnosis is made by the following.

- The history of gritty sore eyes especially in a warm, dry or smoky atmosphere.
- Close inspection, which will reveal reddening of all four lid margins (a kind of blepharitis or blepharopathy).
- Eversion of the lower lids to reveal Meibomianitis, i.e. congested Meibomian glands running at right angles to the lid margins far towards the lower fornix.
- Instillation of eye drops of Rose Bengal, which will show a multiplicity of punctate stains of abnormal conjunctiva overlying the sclera in the exposed area between the eyelids (two triangles with bases at the corneo-scleral junction). The cornea is usually also involved. These eyedrops are rather irritant, especially for dry eyes, and may be preceded by a topical anaesthetic.
- Schirmer's test of tear production, although it is not completely diagnostic, even if repeated. The end of a narrow strip of sterile filter paper is engaged into the lower fornix between the lower lid and conjunctiva overlying the sclera. (Fig. 14.2). After 5 minutes, if tear production is normal, 10 mm or more of the strip will be wetted; less than 5 mm is probably abnormal — especially 0 mm.

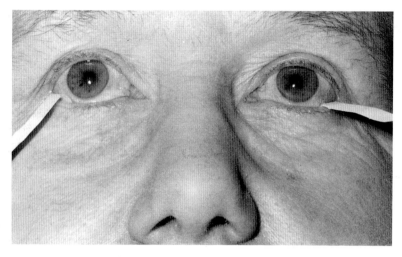

Fig. 14.2. Schirmer test. Strips of sterile filter paper are placed in the lower fornix of conjunctiva. After 5 minutes the length of the strips moistened by tears is measured.

Treatment of dry eyes consists of the regular application of topical artificial tears. There are many different commercial preparations, frequently designed to replace the components of the tear film in approximately similar physiological proportions. The simplest one is Hypromellose eye drops in concentrations of 0.3%, 0.5%, 1% and 2%.

(2) Diminished Secretion of the Mucin Layer
The mucin layer is secreted by goblet cells situated in the conjunctiva. Impairment of mucin secretion may result from conjunctival scarring, usually following chemical burns or autoimmune disease (Stevens–Johnson syndrome and benign mucous membrane pemphigoid) in Western nations, or trachoma in Third World countries.

Treatment consists of replacement with either artifical tears or topical mucomimetic agents.

(3) Impairment of Meibomian Secretion
There are very few clinical disorders in which Meibomian secretion is inadequate for normal requirements, e.g. some forms of blepharitis and the rare situation of severe lid scarring from burns, chemical or otherwise.

The Watering Eye

This may result either from excessive tear secretion (rare) or impairment of tear drainage (common).

Excessive Tear Secretion

Secretion of tears may be reflexly increased in response to stimulation of sensory nerves in either the cornea or conjunctiva, or by emotion. Any noxious stimulus to the cornea or conjunctiva may excite increased tear secretion. The commonest causes are conjunctival or corneal foreign bodies, corneal abrasions, infection of the cornea, and conjunctival infection.

Paradoxically, a dry eye may present occasionally with excessive watering (but see below). Drying of the cornea stimulates sensory nerves within it; this causes reflex increase in tear production from the lacrimal gland, mediated by parasympathetic efferent fibres originating in the salivatory nucleus of the VIIth nerve. The reflex tear production has a higher aqueous component and does not fulfil the lubricating function of the normal tear film. Treatment is by regular topical application of artificial tears, which eliminates the reflex tear production by removal of the predisposing cause.

Reduced Drainage of Tears

Impaired drainage of tears eventually leads to overflow of tears on to the cheek (epiphora) (see Fig. 14.3). Tears normally drain into the lacrimal puncta, easily visible at the medial ends of the upper and lower eyelids. From these puncta, the lacrimal canaliculi pass tears onwards to the lacrimal sac, which is situated in a small bony identation (lacrimal fossa) at the base of the nose near the medial canthus. Tears then pass down the naso-lacrimal duct to reach the inferior meatus of the nose.

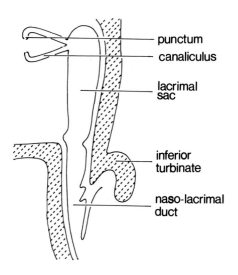

Fig. 14.3. Diagram of coronal section of the right lacrimal drainage system. Congenital obstruction is at the lower end of the naso-lacrimal duct — simple probing usually cures. Epiphora in adults is usually due to permanent obstruction below the lacrimal sac: note that if the lacrimal bone (stippled) adjacent to the sac is removed, flaps of nasal mucosa can be anastomosed to flaps of the lacrimal sac — dacryocystorhinostomy.

The student should watch a 'syringing of the tear passages', commonly performed in adults with topical anaesthesia, in order to confirm or exclude blockage of the tear passages. As a preliminary, a punctum dilator is inserted into the lower canaliculus. Then the tip of a fine lacrimal cannula attached to a syringe filled with sterile saline is inserted just into that canaliculus. The plunger of the syringe is gently depressed. If the tear passages have no obstruction, the patient will taste 'salty water' in the back of the throat. Any complete obstruction beyond the lower canaliculus will prevent access of saline to the nasopharynx, the site being usually at the upper end of the naso-lacrimal duct in adults. Saline will regurgitate through the upper canaliculus.

Systematic consideration is required as follows, however.

(1) *Punctal stenosis.* Narrowing of the lacrimal puncta may occur as a result of chronic inflammation, but usually occurs in the elderly without obvious cause. This is treated by dilatation of the lower punctum with a punctum dilator, or by excision of part of the punctal ring — a 'three-snip' operation.

(2) *Ectropion.* Drainage of tears is obviously dependent on constant apposition of the eyelids (especially their punctum-bearing medial ends) to the anterior surface of the eyeball. The lower punctum accounts for up to 80% of the drainage of tears, the upper punctum and evaporation for the remaining 20%. Surgical correction of the ectropion is usually successful in eliminating the problem. See Fig 12.3.

(3) *Canaliculus blockage.* Obstruction of the lacrimal canaliculi usually results from injury, e.g. by a knife, or occasionally from inflammation. This is treated by a more extensive surgical procedure, often including implantation of silastic tubes within the canaliculi, at least temporarily, to improve canalicular patency; success may well not be achieved.

(4) *Naso-lacrimal duct obstruction.* This is a problem at the extremes of life, either in infancy or in the elderly.

In babies, the naso-lacrimal duct may not fully canalize until the sixth month of life, or even up to the twelfth month, so that surgical correction is not usually performed until 6–12 months of age. The condition is usually simply treated by probing of the duct under general anaesthesia. A repeat probing (or probings) is occasionally necessary.

In the elderly, the obstruction is usually at the upper end of the naso-lacrimal duct just below the lacrimal sac. Probing seldom succeeds. If epiphora is particularly distressing, a dacryocystorhinostomy (DCR) is performed, in which an aperture in the bone between the lacrimal sac and the nose is created; a partial lining of that ostium by mucous membrane is achieved by suturing together flaps fashioned from the nasal mucosa and lacrimal sac. The prognosis for successful cure of epiphora is about 80–90% because late fibrotic blockage of the new passage may occur.

Acute dacryocystitis is sometimes a presenting symptom of obstruction of the nasolacrimal duct in the elderly and occasionally in the baby. Stasis of the contents of the sac is an important factor, sometimes with a preceding mucocele (Fig. 14.4). A red tender swelling appears just below the level of the medial palpebral ligament. (Compare ethmoiditis, which 'points' above that ligament.) A systemic antibiotic may not control the infection quickly enough, so that incision and 'packing' of this abscess of the lacrimal sac is required. When the acute inflammation has settled, and before the antibiotic is withdrawn, *a definitive operation is essential to avoid recurrences*. In the elderly a dacryocystectomy may suffice, usually with surprisingly little complaint from subsequent epiphora, but a dacryocystorhinostomy (DCR) is often possible. In a child, an experienced surgeon can usually achieve a successful DCR, rather than a dacryocystectomy, thereby avoiding a possible lifetime of epiphora.

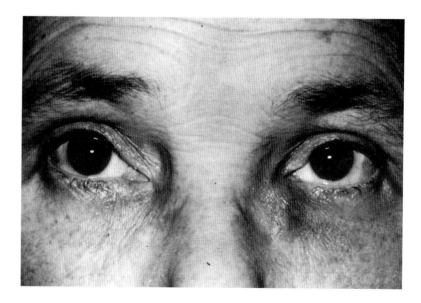

Fig. 14.4. Mucocele of left lacrimal sac due to blockage of the naso-lacrimal duct, often with obstruction of the lacrimal canaliculi. The swelling is below the medial palpebral ligament. An acute dacryocystitis may follow (or arise without preceding mucocele at the same site).

(5) *Nasal passages.* A history of significant disease of the nasal passages should be investigated by an ENT surgeon, because obstruction to the lacrimal system may arise within the nose. Another cause is disease of the maxillary sinus, e.g. carcinoma. *A question about nose-bleeds is essential for all patients with epiphora.*

Chapter 15

TROPICAL OPHTHALMOLOGY

Vitamin A Deficiency and Blinding Malnutrition •
Trachoma
contributed by
John D. C. Anderson

Onchocerciasis • **Leprosy** • **Behçet's Disease**
contributed by
Malcom G. Kerr Muir

Vitamin A Deficiency and Blinding Malnutrition

Doctors know that ... green vegetables, even leaves, make all the difference
between vision and blindness. But rural people and many in the cities are still
unaware of such elementary facts. *Indira Gandhi (1976).*

Acute vitamin A deficiency is the cause of blindness in half of the 1.5
million blind *children* in the world today (WHO estimate), especially in
Asia. Their death rate is high within 1–2 years, mainly because of
susceptibility to infection, which also applies to the 10 million children
with moderate deficiency. There are around 40 million blind people
worldwide.

Clinical Features and Treatment

Retina
Reduced dietary vitamin A (= retinol) causes deficiency of visual
purple (rhodopsin) in retinal rods, so that dark adaptation is poor. The
first symptom is greater difficulty than normal in seeing in dim
illumination, so-called 'night blindness', which is also a feature of
early retinitis pigmentosa (see p. 199). Children's mothers notice that
they are blind after dusk, like domestic chickens which have no rods,
only cones, in their retinae, hence a common local phrase 'chicken
eyes'.

Conjunctiva and Cornea

The next stage is bilateral *dryness* of the conjunctiva and cornea (xerophthalmia), with loss of mucus-secreting goblet cells and conversion of epithelia into a stratified squamous form with keratinization, i.e. the mucous membrane becomes skin-like. An early sign is Bitôt's spots — triangular patches of conjunctiva on each side of the cornea covered with foamy or cheesy material: they are often pigmented and may remain after vitamin A deficiency has disappeared.

Continued severe malnutrition, often aggravated by (acute) diarrhoea or measles, may cause melting away of both corneas (*keratomalacia*) in 24–48 hours until perforation occurs (Fig. 15.1). Aqueous humour escapes and the anterior chamber flattens. Part of the iris usually plugs the gap in the cornea and, when the anterior chamber re-forms, a patch of iris remains adherent to the cornea (anterior synechia). White scar tissue may involve a large area of the cornea (leukoma). In severe cases, the corneal perforation may be so large that the whole eyeball collapses and never re-fills with aqueous humour: a small shrunken residue of the globe remains in the orbit ('phthisis

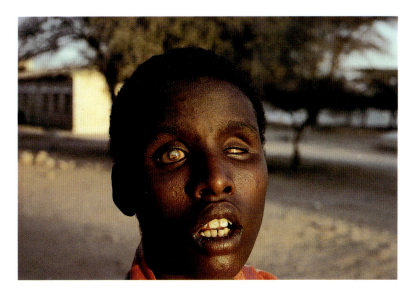

Fig. 15.1. A blind beggar aged 15 years in Somalia. Aged 3 years, his vitamin A deficiency, already producing night blindness, was aggravated by nearly fatal measles which caused keratomalacia. The right cornea shows severe vascularized scarring with a VAR of PL (perception of light). The left cornea had a large perforation resulting in a shrunken eyeball ('phthisis bulbi'): VAL is no PL.

bulbi', which means 'a wasting of the globe', *not* tuberculosis) (Fig. 15.1).

Other Deficiencies
Other deficiencies nearly always co-exist, especially protein-energy malnutrition. These predispose to infections which aggravate deficiencies — a vicious circle.

TREATMENT

Treatment is very urgent.

- 200 000 IU of vitamin A by mouth on two successive days. Or
- In cases of severe gastroenteritis or protein deficiency, 100 000 IU of water-miscible vitamin A intramuscularly, followed by oral vitamin A after 24 hours.
- A protein- and calorie-rich diet.
- Treatment of systemic infections.
- Antibiotic oculentum three times daily.
- If cornea exposed in marasmic infants, carers should close the child's eyelids gently and repeatedly if taping not available.

In Western countries where the common causes of corneal exposure are unconsciousness, due to head injuries or general anaesthesia, and facial paralysis, adhesive tape is usually available to apply to the upper lids to pull them down towards the cheeks (see p. 145). An antibiotic eye ointment is instilled before adhesive taping.

PREVENTION

Prevention has supreme importance. 'Primary health workers' should

- identify the children at risk, especially aged 6 months to 4 years;
- recognize the malnourished ones (mid-arm circumference 12.5 cm or less);
- supply oral vitamin A;
- ensure oral re-hydration in cases of diarrhoea;
- monitor sensible home care of measles.

More general preventive measures are to encourage the home growing *and eating* of dark green leafy vegetables and yellow fruits. Twice-yearly oral vitamin A (200 000 IU) for the 1–5 years group, or the fortification of a universally consumed food such as sugar or tea with a stable and tasteless form of vitamin A is valuable. The prevalence of infection should be reduced, e.g. by improvement of purity of water to prevent diarrhoea and by immunization against measles, pertussis and tuberculosis.

More fundamentally, the problem of poverty remains to be solved.

Trachoma

Trachoma has had a blinding grip on mankind for about five millenia. At present, it affects 400 million people, of whom an estimated 80 million are children with active disease and 6 million are blind. Only by realizing that it is a community disease can we hope to eliminate it.

Scar formation in the eyelids, conjunctiva and cornea, in response to chronic and recurrent infection with Chlamydia trachomatis, is the outstandingly important feature. It is almost invariably bilateral.

Chlamydia trachomatis is a minute atypical bacterium that can grow only inside certain epithelial cells. It has a cell wall, contains both DNA and RNA, and has a limited enzyme system. Only four serotypes (A, B, Ba, C) are associated with endemic trachoma of eye-to-eye transmission; the others (D through K) are associated with conjunctivitis and respiratory infections of the newborn and with infections of the adult urogenital tracts.

This infective agent invades the non-keratinized epithelial cells of the conjunctiva and cornea as rigid-walled *elementary bodies* (EB) 300 nm in diameter. Within hours, DNA transcription leading to RNA and protein synthesis has occurred. The EB is reorganized into a reticulate body that divides many times by binary fission, forming, after 48 hours, an intracytoplasmic inclusion body — a colony of thousands of EBs lying adjacent to the nucleus of the epithelial cell. These can be seen in iodine- or Giemsa-stained conjunctival smears. The host cell then ruptures and thousands more elementary bodies are freed to invade other epithelial cells. Although these bodies may not themselves invade the subepithelial tissues, their toxic metabolic products almost certainly do, and these induce an inflammatory reaction in the cornea, conjunctiva and adjacent tissues. The degree of inflammation and subsequent scarring in trachoma is determined by a combination of (1) the total period of time (months or, more likely, years) in which the individual has been repeatedly reinfected, (2) the size of dose of chlamydia introduced at each reinfection, and (3) the amount of eye damage from other causes such as bacterial and viral infections, or trauma. Prolonged immune responses are responsible for the disastrous scarring of cornea and eyelids and for the resultant physical signs.

EPIDEMIOLOGY

The disease occurs in the 'trachoma belt' — North Africa, the Middle East, the Indian subcontinent and the Far East — but it is also found in parts of southern Europe, in Central and Latin America and among the Australian Aborigines. Its maintenance and spread in a population are encouraged by overcrowding and poor water supply, each contributing to insanitary conditions, e.g. shared and limited water for washing, common cloths for drying and absence of latrines. An additional and escalating factor is the frequently high prevalence of 'eye-seeking' flies, particularly the common house-fly and the smaller *Musca sorbens*, which breeds preferentially on human faeces. These flies, needing moisture and protein (to mature their eggs), move from exposed faeces to the watering eyes and discharging noses of different individuals, and back again indiscriminately (Fig. 15.2). They have been proved to be carriers of both bacteria *and* chlamydia, which explains why the 'fly season' is followed closely by the 'sticky eye season'. Epidemics of mucopurulent *bacterial* conjunctivitis usually occur during the fly season and so, indirectly, enhance reinfection with *Chlamydia trachomatis*. Multiple reinfection with chlamydia, especially if combined with bacterial infection, is the major factor in the development of severe scarring in trachoma.

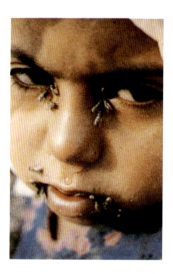

Fig. 15.2. Moisture-seeking flies spread *Chlamydia trachomatis* and other organisms in a dry climate.

SYMPTOMS

In the early stages symptoms range from almost none or a mild bilateral ocular discomfort with a little watering to a severe foreign-body sensation with marked photophobia. If secondary bacterial infection is present, there may be conjunctival hyperaemia, mucopurulent discharge and crusting of the lid margins. When scarring is severe, patients may complain of heaviness of the eyelids, foreign body sensation and blurring of vision. If their eyelashes are turned inwards (trichiasis), irritation and watering are constant. Extensive scarring makes the eyes feel dry. However, the majority of trachoma subjects complain of few symptoms: millions learn to live with their progressive trachoma uncomplainingly.

SIGNS

Conjunctival early signs are best seen on the everted lids, especially the upper lids, with the help of a torch and magnifying loupe. See Fig 11.1 for technique of eversion. Particularly over the upper tarsal plate and in the fornices, lymphoid follicles can be seen, i.e. small (0.2–2 mm diameter), yellowish-white, raised avascular lesions that vary from few to numerous. In severe infections, after weeks or months, these small lesions may become large, yellow and necrotic, and be partially buried in thickened conjunctiva. They represent a cell-mediated specific immune response to the infective agent. The conjunctival membrane becomes thickened by a diffuse cellular infiltration (of neutrophils, lymphocytes, plasma cells and macrophages) and by neo-vascularization. Two very important signs are thus produced: first, the appearance of multiple tiny engorged capillary tufts called *papillae* on the surface of the conjunctiva, which has a red velvety appearance; second, a partial or even complete obscuration of the normally visible conjunctival blood vessels, which indicates a very severe inflammatory reaction. *As the disease progresses, small linear scars or, in more severe cases, large confluent scars appear after some months and are permanent. Contraction of this scar tissue produces the serious complications* (Figs 15.3 and 15.4).

Corneal signs appear first in its *upper* half because of its close contact with the *upper* lid. To see that area of cornea, lift the upper lid and ask the patient to look down as in looking for a corneal foreign body. At first, lesions are so small that a magnifying loupe or slit-lamp micro-scope is required. In long-standing trachoma, the whole cornea may be affected. Epithelial keratitis with tiny shallow ulcers (shown up well with fluorescein staining) is followed by cellular infiltration of the stroma under the infected epithelium. Then, a fibrovascular membrane, called *trachomatous pannus* (Latin 'cloth'), invades the superficial stroma (Fig. 15.3). Follicles are sometimes prominent at the upper limbal region of the cornea; on healing, they leave shallow translucent depressions called *Herbert's pits*, pathognomonic of trachoma.

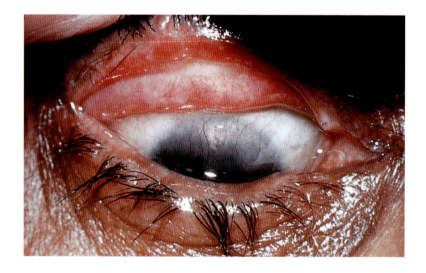

Fig. 15.3. Chronic trachoma. The conjunctival surface of the everted upper lid shows white scar tissue, mainly parallel with the lid margin. That infected surface, in constant contact with the upper cornea, produces typical pannus (vascularized white scar tissue).

External lid signs may be entirely absent. However, some swelling of the lid during the active stage suggests a more severe tarsal infection. The scarring of long-standing trachoma causes the lids to become thickened and in-turned (*entropion*); a few or many lashes may rub against the globe (trichiasis): see Fig. 15.4; the lid aperture may be widened from scarring of the lid retractor muscles, or the lid margins may become notched from scarring. A defect in lid-closure may result, noticeable when the patient blinks or is asked to close the eyes gently as in sleep.

COMPLICATIONS

Complications are all the result of scarring. In the cornea it causes blurring of vision directly by central corneal opacities and indirectly by distorting the corneal curvature (irregular astigmatism: see p. 26). Figs. 15.3 and

15.4. The cornea's resistance to secondary infection is reduced by two factors: first, the constant trauma of the in-turned lashes of trichiasis (Fig. 15.4); second, inadequate wetting by tears. The latter results partly from failure to produce mucin by conjunctival goblet-cells destroyed by scarring, and partly from blockage of the ducts of tear producing glands, but also simply from mechanical failure of a distorted and contracted eyelid to sweep an even tear film over the cornea. A compromised cornea is always at risk of bacterial or other infection so that corneal ulceration leading to suppurative keratitis is one of the pathways to blindness in chronic trachoma.

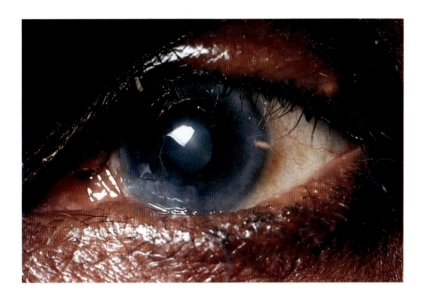

Fig. 15.4. Trichiasis (distortion of eyelashes) resulting from contraction of fibrous tissue excited by chronic trachoma. The eyelashes rub on the cornea, hence (peripheral) corneal opacities with vascularization. Cataract also present. VAL 3/36.

COMMUNITY SIGNS

In some areas of endemic trachoma, blindness is rare: 'non-blinding trachoma'. In others with endemic, or rather hyperendemic, trachoma, blindness is relatively common: 'blinding trachoma'. In the latter areas, poverty, large families, overcrowding, poor water supply, lack of hygiene and many flies are typical, so that repeated re-infections with chlamydia and bacteria occur. The difference between these two communities is not due to any difference in strains of *Chlamydia*. Treatment on a *community*, rather than on an individual, basis is indicated; see below.

Treatment

Within about 10 days, antibiotics can make an individual chlamydia-free, because they prevent multiplication of the agent within the epithelial cells which are routinely shed from the surface within that period. Where the conjunctiva is severely disorganized, treatment is required for several weeks. The signs may take three months to disappear.

Both of the following, alone or together, are effective. (1) Oral sulphonamide, e.g. triple sulpha for 3 weeks or a long-acting drug such as sulphametopyrazine (30 mg/kg) at one dose per week for 3 weeks. The risks of sulphonamide complications, e.g. the rare Stevens–Johnson syndrome, must be considered. Alternatively, *oral* tetracycline 250 mg four times daily, or doxycycline 100 mg daily, for 3 weeks is effective, but tetracycline is not advised for children or pregnant women because of yellowing of developing teeth; for them erythromycin may be substituted. (2) Topical oculentum tetracycline 1% three times daily for 6 weeks.

Surgical treatment of the lid deformities is necessary for three reasons: first, to reduce the risk of blinding complications such as corneal ulceration; secondly, to relieve the patient's physical discomfort; and thirdly, to make the eye less watery and less attractive to eye-seeking flies.

Mild trichiasis is often treated by simple epilation, which must be repeated since the distorted lashes grow again. Electrolysis of individual lashes may succeed in a localized area of trichiasis, but is difficult and unpleasant. Cryotherapy is a more satisfactory method. See also p. 146. Many useful operations have been devised to correct cicatricial entropion of the upper and lower eyelids. Great vigilance is required to diagnose exposure keratitis, which needs careful treatment (p. 145). Corneal grafting is often unsuccessful because of the vascularity of the host cornea (see p. 122), and because of the difficulty in maintaining good aftercare, including topical corticosteroid immunosuppressives; the resulting host – graft reaction often causes opacification of the graft.

TREATMENT OF THE COMMUNITY

The continuing pressure of transmission of infection from the 'ocular community pool' of *Chlamydia trachomatis*, constantly topped up by multiple infected persons, especially children, who re-infect each other, makes individual treatment disappointing. Methods of breaking the cycles of reinfection, and of reducing the community concentration of chlamydia must be emphasized. Just as transmission of AIDS could be greatly reduced by eliminating promiscuity, so trachoma could be eliminated or reduced by attacking transmission points. Trachoma was a serious public health problem 150 years ago in Europe, where it flourished in conditions of poverty and overcrowding. But, 50 years before antibiotics were discovered, it had vanished with improved prosperity, new laws on housing, piped water, adequate sewage disposal and better hygiene. The most important preventive measures are

- a plentiful water-supply, e.g. by well-digging;
- health education to the community, especially school children, particularly on regular face-washing;
- fly-control measures; and, related to that,
- the provision and clean use of latrines;
- increased birth interval by family planning to reduce the population density of small children living close together who collect and multiply chlamydia and shed them to others;
- drug treatment on a mass scale to all children under 10 years, but especially to pre-school children, in order to reduce the ocular reservoir of chlamydia in the community. One regimen recommended by WHO is to give oculentum tetracycline to school children twice daily every day for one week per month for six months. There are several other equally effective regimens.

In a refugee camp of 60 000 people in Somalia, a survey found a high prevalence of active trachoma described as a 'forest fire'. Fifteen refugee community health workers and one Somali nurse carried out a simple programme. They combined a face- and hand-washing programme among school and pre-school children with a once-daily instillation of 3% tetracycline eye ointment. Some fly control was also attempted. The results was impressive. A second survey showed a reduction of active trachoma to *one-third* of its previous level.

The lesson? *Blinding trachoma is a community problem* that could be rapidly controlled by highly motivated community action.

Onchocerciasis

Onchocerciasis is a potentially blinding disease caused by the filarial worm *Onchocerca volvulus* transmitted by the blackfly (*Simulium* species), which occurs in Central and South America, equatorial Africa and the

Yemen. Blindness results from direct involvement of the optic nerve, chorioretina and cornea and from glaucoma and cataract secondary to long-standing iritis.

EPIDEMIOLOGY

Of the estimated 50 million infected persons, one million are blind, with many more severely disabled. Blindness is related to the microfilarial load, which in turn depends on the intensity and duration of transmission. The devastation for the individual is compounded for the community because the blindness affects the young working population. The voracious biting habit of the flies, in addition to their capacity as vectors, has rendered many fertile riverine areas uninhabitable.

Man is the definitive host and reservoir of this microfilarial load produced continually by adult female worms that can survive for up to 15 years in the human body. These microfilariae reside principally in the skin, but also occur in the kidneys, blood and cerebrospinal fluid.

During a blood-meal of the female blackfly, microfilariae gain access to this intermediate host where they continue their development. Thus, disease patterns depend on *Simulium* behaviour. One important characteristic is the need for well-oxygenated running water at its breeding sites, which thus provide identifiable and reasonably circumscribed areas for vector control programmes.

CLINICAL FEATURES

Several years elapse before the disease becomes manifest, most obviously in the skin as a chronic pruritic eruption leading to atrophy, depigmentation and loss of elasticity, and as subcutaneous nodules which represent coiled masses of adult worms.

The overriding morbidity relates to the ocular consequences of microfilarial infestation. These have been identified histologically in all ocular tissues, and clinically may be seen with a slit-lamp microscope in the cornea, anterior chamber (where the numbers seen can be increased by rubbing the patient's eyes or putting the head between the legs just prior to examination), and the vitreous.

Examination of skin and conjunctival biopsies may show numerous motile microfilariae, which may provide a route of entry to the eye, but it is likely that they also enter along the posterior ciliary vessels and nerves and possibly the cerebrospinal fluid.

The live parasite excites no inflammatory response. However, death of the parasite or release of its antigens, whether natural or due to drugs, generates a localized inflammatory response that often damages the host tissues. The pattern of disease in onchocerciasis is thus determined by the nature of the host's immune response to parasite death.

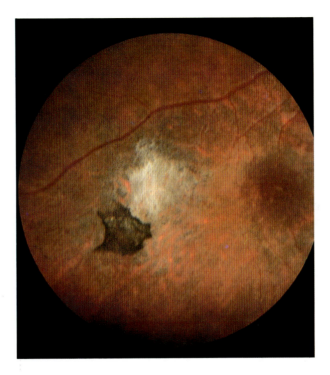

Fig. 15.5. Onchocerciasis. A focus of hyperpigmentation lies near an area of white scar tissue; larger choroidal vessels have become visible around them. Fortunately in this mild case or early stage of quiescent (healed) choroidoretinal inflammation, the macula has been spared (dark red circle on right of the picture).

- *Conjunctiva.* A mild conjunctivitis occurs, particularly following treatment. Recurrent disease may produce hyperpigmentation.
- *Cornea.* Typically, after early exposure and in mildly infected individuals, a localized inflammatory response leads to a punctate (snowflake) keratitis which usually resolves completely. This represents immediate hypersensitivity, in contrast to a sclerosing keratitis which occurs in those individuals with a high microfilarial load and impaired cell-mediated immunity. A chronic low-grade keratitis ensues with the development of pannus and stromal disease with progressive opacification. It is possible that different parasite

strains as well as the variable immune response contribute to the patterns of clinical disease.

- *Anterior uvea.* An insidious iridocyclitis, often complicated by iris atrophy, posterior synechiae and secondary glaucoma, is an invariable part of the disease and a major contributor to visual impairment.
- *Choroid and retina.* There is a spectrum of disease from mild pigment epithelial atrophy, initially only demonstrable by fluorescein angiography, through discrete areas of atrophy of retina and underlying choriocapillaris revealing the larger choroidal vessels (Fig. 15.5), to large areas of posterior polar atrophy often with foci of hyperpigmentation.
- *Optic nerve.* A large proportion of blindness is due to inflammatory disease of the optic nerve, resulting in widespread loss of visual field, compounding the already impaired acuity due to chorioretinal atrophy. Initially there is a papillitis that resolves into segmental and ultimately total optic atrophy, with corresponding defects in the nerve fibre bundle layer.

Management

Individual
Until recently the anthelmintics active against adult and microfilarial worms were complicated by severe sight-threatening and general reactions, which limited their use and required close medical supervision. However, ivermectin, principally a microfilaricide, does not induce ocular side-effects; serious systemic side-effects, such as transient postural hypotension, bronchospasm in asthmatics and a bullous skin eruption, are rare. Although it does not kill the adult worm, an effect upon its uterus reduces the microfilarial load. The other remarkable feature of ivermectin is its infrequent dosage, e.g. a single oral dose that may have to be repeated every three months to maintain low microfilarial levels. Excision of skin nodules (which contain adult worms), particularly in the head region, is advocated.

The Community
Community programmes are essential to break the cycle of transmission and to remove the reservoir of microfilariae. Long-term vector control programmes using biodegradeable insecticides targeted to the riverine breeding sites are in operation. Education programmes should concentrate on means of reducing exposure to *Simulium* breeding sites and use of protective clothing.

Leprosy

Leprosy is a chronic infective disease of neural tissue caused by *Mycobacterium leprae*, a slowly multiplying organism which thrives in cooler environments so that it preferentially affects superficial tissues. Transmission is principally by droplet spread from the nasal mucosa. It is estimated that at least 15 million people are affected, of whom 750 000 are blind. The disease is associated with overcrowding and poor hygiene; climate is *not* an important limiting factor.

PATHOGENESIS

An individual's response to exposure to *M. leprae* has racial variations but depends mainly on the type of immunological reaction that follows the initial bacteraemia. A brisk cell-mediated response results in a tuberculoid lesion in which bacilli are rarely found, whilst lepromatous lesions are associated with minimal inflammatory reaction but numerous bacilli. There is a great spectrum of disease between these two groups.

CLINICAL FEATURES (see Fig. 15.6)

There are three distinct pathways to blindness in leprosy, all primarily involving the anterior segment:

● facial and trigeminal nerve disease;
● hypersensitivity reactions;
● direct bacillary invasion of the globe.

Facial and Trigeminal Nerve Disease
In their superficial course, these nerves are susceptible to leprous invasion, resulting in weakness of the orbicularis oculi muscle, which leads to deficient blinking, inadequate tear film, lower lid ectropion, poor lid closure (see Fig. 15.6) and exposure keratitis. Scarring of skin contributes. Deficient tear drainage due to ectropion or leprous involvement of the naso-lacrimal duct leads to an accumulation of infected debris, which may contribute to a suppurative keratitis and rapid disorganization of the cornea. Trigeminal disease results in impaired corneal sensation.

Hypersensitivity Reactions
The immune complex hypersensitivity response known as erythema nodosum leprosum with cutaneous, renal and joint components is often

associated with an exudative iritis and scleritis that may be complicated by anterior and/or posterior synechiae and may lead to secondary glaucoma.

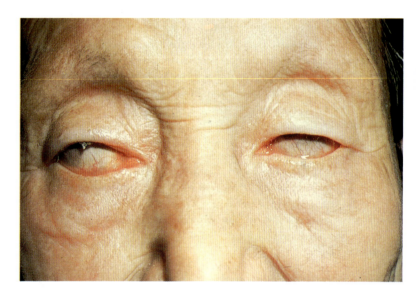

Fig. 15.6. Lepromatous leprosy. Failure on attempted eyelid closure (lagophthalmos). The eyeballs normally turn upwards on lid closure, an associated (protective) reflex.

Direct Invasion of Ocular Tissue
This occurs in lepromatous disease and more often in temperate climates, producing a keratitis, scleritis or iritis.

Corneal Disease (Keratitis)
An asymptomatic fine punctate subepithelial infiltrate beginning in the upper temporal quadrant is the initial manifestation of involvement of the corneal nerves, which may become beaded and calcified owing to aggregations of phagocytosed bacilli. Progression to other quadrants or deep stroma may occur, but pannus is unusual unless accompanied by limbal granulomata. A sclerosing keratitis may be associated with leprous episcleritis or scleritis, while band keratopathy is a common feature of chronic iritis.

Uveal Disease
While acute iritis may occur in all forms of leprosy, chronic iritis is limited to the lepromatous form in which there is a heavy bacillary

invasion of the anterior uvea, whose temperature is some $3\,^\circ$C less than body temperature, and contains numerous non-myelinated nerve fibres, the ideal conditions for multiplication.

Insidiously progressive, the mild iritis is associated in its early stages with discrete yellow globular deposits within the iris stroma (iris pearls) which gradually protrude and eventually fall into the anterior chamber — these are aggregates of phagocytosed bacilli within mononuclear cells.

With time there is progressive iris atrophy, marked miosis and little response to mydriatic drugs. The miosis in combination with axial corneal or lens opacities contributes greatly to the visual handicap and appears to result from preferential involvement of the dilator muscle. Posterior synechiae are not a feature of this neuroparalytic iritis but a floccular post-inflammatory membrane may occlude the pupil or produce pupil block glaucoma.

Diffuse lepromatous disease also affects the skin appendages, e.g. loss of eyebrows is a common and often socially debilitating sequel.

Management

The principal aim is the interruption of the cycle of transmission by using drugs, hitherto as long-term regimens but more recently as shorter multidrug therapies — rifampicin, dapsone and clofazimine.

The aim is often thwarted by the social stigma that accompanies this disease, whereby patients are identified by limb and facial deformities. This has three main effects:

- Patients become outcasts from their own communities.
- Patients are often reluctant to seek advice for fear of a diagnosis of leprosy and so often present late in the disease with established neurological deficit.
- In many countries medical and paramedical personnel are reluctant to treat leprosy.

Early identification of patients within the context of primary health care should be followed by careful surveillance.

While the acute iritis should be treated with topical steroids and mydriatics, it is doubtful whether steroids have any useful role in chronic iritis, but pupil dilatation using sympathomimetic drugs such as phenylephrine may be beneficial in reducing the incapacitating miosis.

Lid deformities require plastic surgical repair. If there is impaired corneal sensation, the patient and his relatives are instructed to examine the eye daily for evidence of impaired vision or redness of the eye and to seek urgent medical attention.

Leprosy is an eminently treatable disease. Many patients do not receive treatment because of social prejudice. The challenge therefore is to overcome this stigma, achieve earlier diagnosis and treatment, and thereby prevent deformity and blindness.

Behçet's Syndrome

Behçet's syndrome is a multisystem disease whose aetiology is unknown. An immune complex-mediated vasculitis, possibly related to release of retinal-S antigen, is the common pathological event. All parts of the eye may be involved and vision becomes severely impaired owing to the consequences of recurrent uveitis and widespread ischaemic retinal vasculitis.

EPIDEMIOLOGY

The condition is more common in Japan and the Eastern Mediterranean and tends to affect young adult men more than women. There is a strong association, particularly in Japan, between ocular disease and HLA-B5 antigen.

CLINICAL FEATURES

For diagnostic and investigational protocols, the syndrome has been subdivided on the basis of the common signs into major and minor criteria.

Major: 1. aphthous ulceration
        2. genital ulceration
        3. skin lesions
        4. any ocular manifestation
Minor: 1. arthritis/synovitis
        2. gastrointestinal disorder
        3. epididymitis
        4. meningo-encephalitis

PRESENTATION

Aphthous Ulcers
The majority of patients present with oral or genital ulceration. These painful lesions may be single but more often occur in crops. They are sharply demarcated with a yellow base and a red areola and may remain

indolent, often taking several months to heal. They do not scar. Rarely, oesophageal lesions may produce severe dysphagia. Genital ulcers occur on the scrotum and the labia majora.

Cutaneous vasculitis. Skin manifestations are common with a variety of presentations, from pustules to nodules which may resemble erythema nodosum. During active disease, pustules may occur at injection sites.

Thrombophlebitis, often of larger vessels, is common.

The *neurological* features of a meningo-encephalitis are very variable from mild meningism to specific localizing signs or even a confusional state.

Ocular signs. 80% of patients have ocular signs which are commoner and more severe in males. *Uveitis:* Recurrent episodes of acute combined anterior and posterior uveitis may resolve but the majority progress to chronic indolent uveitis complicated by cataract and glaucoma. *Retina:* Several disease patterns occur, all of which are manifestations of an ischaemic vasculitis. A diffuse vascular leakage may lead to chronic macular and disc oedema. Retinal phlebitis may lead to ischaemic branch or central retinal vein occlusion that may induce neovascularization followed by vitreous haemorrhage. Extensive retinal vascular disease is followed by retinal and pigment epithelial atrophy and finally secondary optic atrophy.

Management

Behçet's syndrome has an unpredictable course. Cytotoxic agents (azathioprine, cyclophosphamide, chlorambucil) in combination with steroids reduce the rate of relapse and probably the severity of ulcerative and ocular disease. The non-cytotoxic immune modulator cyclosporin A with its selective action against T-helper cells induces immuno-suppression, which has been beneficial. Given the intensity of the leukocytic infiltration in the vasculitis, the use of colchicine as an inhibitor of chemotaxis and leukocyte lysosomal enzyme release has also been advocated. These drugs have serious side-effects and the management of such patients with complicated treatment regimens requires careful medical supervision.

Chapter 16

GENETICS IN OPHTHALMOLOGY

The principles of genetics apply to ophthalmology just as elsewhere in medicine and biology. Conversely, some knowledge of hereditary eye diseases will help the student to appreciate aspects of genetics in general. Relatively common inherited eye diseases (see p. 208) are briefly considered in this chapter so that the practitioner can provide explanation and guidance for some of his patients and their families. For basic genetics, the readers should consult appropriate texts.

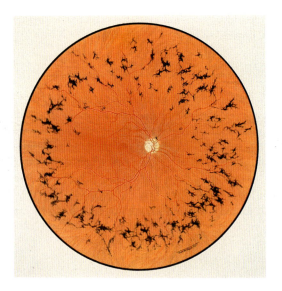

Fig. 16.1. Retinitis pigmentosa (not an inflammation of the retina, in spite of the name). Note the 'bone-corpuscle' pattern of equatorial (mid-peripheral) pigmentation, which often obscures retinal vessels: this hereditary retinal degeneration spreads slowly anteriorly and posteriorly. The retinal vessels are thin and the optic disc is pale.

Retinitis Pigmentosa

Retinitis pigmentosa (RP) is a poor name for a group of diseases with a very similar clinical picture that affects 1 in 5000 of the population. See Fig. 16.1. 'Primary pigmentary degeneration' of the retina is little better. A 'retinal dystrophy' is rather non-specific so that 'tapeto-retinal dystrophy' is sometimes employed. The disease is bilaterally symmetrical, a feature of genetic disease in general. Ophthalmoscopically, pigmentation is seen first in the mid-periphery of the fundus, with a pattern like 'bone-corpuscles', which is associated with degeneration of the retinal receptors in that area (mainly rods, hence greater difficulty than usual in seeing in dull illumination, so-called 'night blindness'). A characteristic of the pigment is that it often obscures the retinal vessels.

A ring scotoma (blind area) in the mid-periphery of the field ensues. See Fig. 16.2. The degeneration with pigmentation and the ring scotoma spread anteriorly and posteriorly until only a small central field remains — 'tunnel vision' is a lay term often used for this disease (the end-stages of the glaucomas often show the same field loss). The visual acuity late in the disease may still be 6/6, but the loss of all the peripheral field makes the patient effectively blind because he cannot move around safely — he lacks 'navigational vision'.

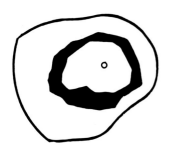 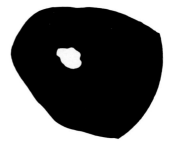

Fig. 16.2. Fields of vision in retinitis pigmentosa. Accompanied by 'night blindness', i.e. greater difficulty than normal in seeing in dull illumination, a mid-peripheral scotoma first appears — a dense irregular black ring in the left diagram (left eye): the small central ring indicates the centre of the field (fixation point). The right diagram (right eye) shows an advanced case with only a small intact area of residual central field — 'tunnel vision' or 'tube field'. Almost invariably both eyes are affected and the progression is equal.

In this disease, pedigrees show any of the three Mendelian routes — autosomal recessive (AR), autosomal dominant (AD) and X-linked recessive (XLR), the commonest being the first, which has an early onset and is quickly progressive. The X-linked form behaves rather similarly but the AD form usually starts later in adult life and is very slowly progressive. The female carrier of the X-linked form shows a mild form of the disease with mild ophthalmoscopic signs, as would be expected from the Lyon principle: random suppression of one X chromosome in the cells of the female.

Most examples of RP present as sporadic cases, i.e. with no previous family history, which applies to many hereditary diseases. The majority of these are probably due to recessive genes. *Enquiry about consanguinity of parents is often forgotten in taking a family history, but is very important in all cases.* A small proportion of sporadic cases may turn out to represent dominant mutations. If the sporadic case is male, then the possibility of X-linkage must be carefully considered. (One of the possible two X-linked RP genes has been mapped to the region of the L1.28 marker in the short arm of the X chromosome, quite near the centromere.) *A very important characteristic of an X-linked pedigree is that there must be no case of male-to-male transmission,* for which a search must be specifically made; an AD pedigree will be expected, of course, to show one or more examples of male-to-male transmission.

A small proportion of families with RP have other associated diseases, e.g. deafness (Usher's syndrome: AR), polydactyly (Bardet–Biedl syndrome: AR), abetalipoproteinaemia (AR).

Point mutations in the gene encoding rhodopsin (3q) have been found in some families with dominant RP. Rhodopsin is the light-sensitive pigment in rods, which predominate in the peripheral retina (compare cones, which predominate in the macular area, particularly the fovea). The first to be found was a cytosine-to-adenine mutation in codon 23 of the rhodopsin gene in 3q. That dictates a change from proline to histidine at the 23rd amino acid from the amino terminus in the rhodopsin molecule itself.

Various other mutations have subsequently been identified, often with a fairly characteristic retinal dysfunction if assessed by subtle tests.

Beware Recessive Genes

When a sporadic case of an hereditary or possibly hereditary disease presents, especially in a newborn child, the possibility or indeed probability of autosomal recessive disease should be considered. Many tragic families exist in which a second affected child has been born because no warning had been given to the parents after the first affected child. An example concerns Leber's congenital amaurosis; this should not be confused with Leber's hereditary (optic) neuroretinopathy (LHON), which is described later in this chapter. An affected child is usually born blind (which is not easy to diagnose) but there are no abnormalities visible ophthalmoscopically: however, the electro-retinogram is 'flat' and that is often required to make the diagnosis. The firstborn in Fig. 16.3 was not finally realized to be blind until 2 years of age, partly because the mother insisted on repeat examinations. Probably the diagnosis of Leber's congenital amaurosis was made then, but no genetic information was given to the parents. The second-born child was soon diagnosed as blind also and the necessary genetic information was belatedly given — a 1-in-4 chance of the disease in any future children of that couple, irrespective of how many affected or unaffected preceded a birth. Families with autosomal recessive disease should be warned of their greater risk of reappearance of the disease if they pair consanguineously. However, they can be reassured that a random association outside their parents' families results in only a slightly greater risk of their disease in their children than in a random association between any two non-consanguineous individuals in the population at large.

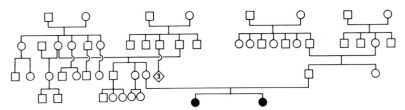

Fig. 16.3. Leber's congenital amaurosis (= blindness), the commonest cause of blindness at birth or an early age, which, however, is fortunately very rare. Note the 'horizontal' pattern of the pedigree, i.e. only one generation is affected, typical of autosomal recessive (AR) inheritance. The second blind child was a preventable tragedy, but no counselling was given on the first diagnosis. □ Normal male; ○ normal female; ● affected female.

Note that a typical feature of a pedigree with recessive disease is a 'horizontal' pattern, i.e. only one generation is affected. Compare the 'vertical' pattern in autosomal dominant disease, in which affected individuals are found in two or more successive generations. Approximately 25% of a sibship will be affected in AR disease. The family in Fig. 16.3 is particularly tragic because 100% have been affected: in small families quite often none will be affected, of course.

A germ-line mutation producing a dominant disease will simulate a recessive inheritance in the first generation (parents somatically unaffected although one has mutated germ cells), but the affected individuals will have a 50% risk of passing on the disease.

Retinoblastoma

Retinoblastoma is of great genetic interest. Clinically it presents usually because the mother notices a whitish or grey appearance in one (or occasionally both) pupils, at first only from certain angles. It may present as a squint (because of reduced vision in one eye), which explains one reason why ophthalmologists examine both fundi of squinting children as soon as possible. It is a highly malignant tumour of retinal receptors of children usually under 2½ years, often under 6–12 months, but seldom over 5 years. It spreads quickly into the optic nerve directly, and metastatically to the liver and lungs. Often it is bilateral. An independent tumour may arise in the pineal gland — the third eye — in the vestigial retinal receptors there ('trilateral retinoblastoma'). A very high proportion of survivors will develop tumours elsewhere, especially osteogenic sarcoma of femur, by the age of 40 years.

It is hereditary. The empirical risk to siblings and children of a unilateral sporadic case is about 4%. Although a bilateral case has almost a 50% chance of passing the disease on to his or her children (and *usually* has an affected parent) the disease is actually recessive. Knudson devised his 'two-hit' hypothesis to explain the genetics of the so-called 'retinoblastoma gene' which, when functioning normally, is an anti-oncogene. The disease is recessive because two abnormal genes (in chromosome 13) are required to produce a neoplastic cell. One abnormal gene is usually inherited — the first 'hit', usually in a paternally-derived chromosome. By chance, a somatic mutation (or non-disjunctional loss, or a deletion, etc.) is quite likely to occur in a maternally or paternally derived chromosome in one or more of the millions of actively developing retinal receptors, in which case that cell or these cells, lacking *both* normal forms of this particular anti-oncogene, will become malignant. That somatic occurrence is the second 'hit'. Even when one or two patches of tumour have been treated successfully (by cryotherapy, radiotherapy or radioactive plaque on the surface of the sclera), regular examination under anaesthesia every few weeks is required until the age of about 5 years. If diagnosis is early, enucleation can usually be avoided; fortunately, bilateral enucleation is rarely indicated.

Congenital Glaucoma

(See p. 65.) Congenital glaucoma is probably AR with incomplete penetrance (i.e. some homozygotes are unaffected) so that the risk to future siblings is about 1 in 8; males are more often affected than females. The cause is residual neural crest tissue in the angle of the anterior chamber, hence the usual operative treatment of goniotomy, in which a knife-needle is slid across the anterior chamber under gonioscopic control with an operation microscope, and this abnormal tissue is incised. An alternative name *buphthalmos* (literally, 'the eye of an ox') describes the enlarged eyeball resulting from a rise in intraocular pressure in babies, which cannot occur in adults. The child presents constantly crying with pain in the eyes, and with eyelids tightly shut because of photophobia: these symptoms require emergency referral to an eye specialist, whatever the cause might turn out to be (e.g. bilateral conjunctivitis is possible).

Congenital Cataract
Usually bilateral, congenital cataract presents in most cases with a white pupil as seen from any direction. Most cases are sporadic and presumptively AR but there is a 12% chance or more that such a case will pass the disease on to children, i.e. a dominant mutation has occurred. Many AD families have been described.

Aniridia
Meaning congenital (bilateral) absence of iris, aniridia is often complicated by glaucoma because of anomalies in the angle of the anterior chamber, and cataract, with a poor ultimate prognosis for vision. It is inherited as a dominant trait — gene in 11p. The mutation rate is quite high. Again an anti-oncogene is involved. Four conditions are associated: Wilm's tumour (nephroblastoma), Aniridia, Genito-urinary abnormalities and/or mental Retardation, the WAGR syndrome.

Subluxated Lenses
These may be congenital and restricted to the eyes (AR). More often they are part of Marfan syndrome (tall stature, wider arm span than height, long thin fingers and coarctation of aorta and other cardiovascular diseases), which is AD. The common feature is a defect in fibrillin, which is a protein in elastic tissue, due to a defect in a gene at 15q 21.1.

Mitochondrial Inheritance
Leber's hereditary neuroretinopathy, or optic neuropathy (LHON), although rare, has long been known to show an unusual pattern in pedigrees: the affected or carrier male *never* passes on the disease to *any* subsequent generation, while the affected or carrier female passes on the disease or the carrier state to *all* her children. For some unknown reason, not all carriers develop the disease and there is a preponderance in males. Compare with X-linked heredity.

The disease presents usually around the twenties, with decreasing visual acuity to 6/60 or less in one eye, followed by the other, over a period of a month or so; field charting shows a central scotoma. In a few cases, some recovery takes place. Telangiectasis of fine blood vessels around the optic discs may regress as the disease progresses to atrophy; in the early stages slight papilloedema is often present. Cardiovascular abnormalities are common in carriers and affected individuals in these families, especially the Wolff–Parkinson–White syndrome with a short PR interval, a long QRS complex of >0.1 second and an extra delta wave; subsarcolemmal 'ragged red fibres' are often found on histology of muscles.

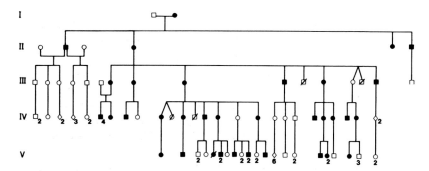

Fig. 16.4. Pedigree of family with Leber's hereditary optic neuroretinopathy (LHON) showing characteristics of mitochondrial (cytoplasmic) inheritance. Affected females (●) transmit the disease or carrier state to *all* children, male or female: note two unaffected but transmitting carrier females III,13 and IV,16. *No male transmits the disease or carrier state to any male or female in any future generation* (compare X-linked disease). ■ , ● = affected male, female; / = deceased; □ , ○ = unaffected male, female; ◇ = unaffected male or female. Numbers indicated in sibship, if more than one. (Reprinted from Wallace, D.C. *Brain* **93**, 121–132, 1970, by permission of Oxford University Press).

The typical family history will support the diagnosis. See Fig. 16.4. Sporadic cases occur, in whom the differential diagnosis will include multiple sclerosis, intracranial — especially pituitary — tumour, and tobacco – alcohol amblyopia; 80% of MS patients show oligoclonal banding on protein electrophoresis of CSF, and magnetic resonance imaging (MRI) brain scanning shows lesions throughout the white matter. Particularly in sporadic cases, the highly specific tests mentioned below would often establish the diagnosis.

The cause of the disease in a substantial proportion of cases is a mutation from the normal guanine to abnormal adenine at position 11 778 in the mitochondrial DNA (mtDNA, which has had all of its 16 569 bases sequenced). That mutation results in a deficiency in the respiratory enzyme NADH dehydrogenase, subunit 4, in which the normal 340th amino acid, arginine, is replaced by the 'pathological' histidine. Mitochondrial DNA exists in the form of *double rings* in the large amount of cytoplasm of the ovum and the small amount of cytoplasm of the sperm. However, at fertilization the sperm adds only its nuclear DNA to the ovum, jettisoning its small amount of cytoplasm with all its mtDNA outside the ovum. *Accordingly the male's sperm cannot transmit his LHON or, of course, the carrier state.* Conversely, since any child, male or female, is dependent on the mother's mtDNA for 13 out of 67 of his respiratory enzymes (54 are coded by nuclear DNA), all the children of an affected or carrier mother will acquire the trait that may (especially in males) or may not (especially in females) cause the full-blown disease.

A *deletion* in the mtDNA is a cause of the more rare Kearns – Sayre syndrome (extraocular muscle dystrophy, especially with ptosis, generalized muscle weakness — again with 'ragged red fibres' on histology of muscle biopsy — and a pigmentary retinopathy like retinitis pigmentosa, and complete heart block), which tends to occur only in sporadic cases because the patients seldom procreate.

Other very rare diseases of genetic interest with similar causes are the MELAS (Mitochondrial Encephalomyopathy, Lactic Acidosis and Stroke-like episodes) and the MERRF (Myoclonic Epilepsy with Ragged Red Fibres) syndromes.

The diagnosis can be established biochemically in LHON by the application of SfaN1, a restriction enzyme which cuts mtDNA if the normal guanine is present in the mtDNA but will not cut at that site if the abnormal adenine is present; hence on electrophoresis there will be smaller faster-and-further-moving fragments in the former, normal, case but larger slower-and-shorter-moving fragments in the latter, abnormal case. A complementary radioactive probe reveals the abnormal band. Conversely, Mae III, another restriction enzyme, cuts the mtDNA if the mutation adenine *is* present but not if the normal base is present. Two provisos exist. About 50% of cases or families have fairly typical LHON that is due to one of several *other* possible mutations for which these tests would not give positive results. Secondly, different patients in families and different tissues in patients show heteroplasmy, i.e. a variable proportion of the mtDNA double rings harbour the mutation, the remainder being normal, so that several affected and unaffected members of a family should be examined and several tissues (blood cells, skin, muscle biopsies, etc.) from any suspected patient should be examined.

Social Considerations

BLIND MARRYING THE BLIND

Although efforts are being made to integrate the handicapped into normal society, there are difficulties. Schools and workshops, with sexes mixed, for the blind, deaf, etc., are probably unavoidable. A high proportion in blind schools have hereditary diseases, often AR but not seldom AD and XLR. It is not surprising that pairing between blind persons occurs: the bond of shared affliction must be strong. Usually, for example when the couple have different AR diseases, there is little risk of blindness in the children, although the parents and children have difficult social problems for the whole of their lifetimes. If both parents have the identical AR disease, 100% of the children will be blind. If both parents have blinding AD disease(s), there is a 75% risk of blindness for any child.

GENETIC COUNSELLING

These few examples from ophthalmology have their counterpart in every other area of medicine. Affected families should be given information to allow the individuals to decide for themselves whether to risk imposing their handicap on their children — which risk they surprisingly often decide to take, so powerful is the procreative instinct, which should be differentiated from the sex instinct.

Chapter 17

EPIDEMIOLOGY OF VISUAL LOSS

The most important aspect in approaching any new subject is to ensure an adequate sense of perspective. The relative probability of different diagnoses is dependent upon many factors, of which the most relevant to ophthalmology are probably geographical location and age.

Geographical Location

It is difficult for inhabitants of Western nations to comprehend fully the diseases causing blindness in Third World countries, as those problems simply do not exist in the developed world to any significant degree. At least 40 million people are estimated to be blind worldwide; most of these patients live in the Third World, and, tragically, many are suffering from preventable or treatable conditions. The commonest causes of blindness worldwide are infection (particularly trachoma) and malnutrition (especially xerophthalmia). These conditions are considered in detail in Chapter 15, but it is essential for the student to appreciate that these initially innocuous conditions, which require merely a brief description in a medical textbook and which are totally preventable by simple treatment, are responsible for a significant proportion of world blindness, and the unimaginable suffering inevitably associated with this condition. Lack of available surgical skills also condemns many in poor countries to treatable blindness from cataract.

Prevalence of Blindness in England

In the most recent year for which statistics are available, around 1 in 500 of the population was 'registered blind' (p. 8). In each of the previous five years, about 1 in 3000 of the population was newly registered blind; of these, 76% were over 64 years of age, the majority (62%) being female. Additionally, about 1 in 4500 were registered 'partially sighted' (p. 8) annually.

The commonest reasons for new blind registrations for all ages were:

Macular degeneration	37%	
Glaucoma	12.5%	
Cataract	8.8%	
Diabetic retinopathy	8%	(the commonest cause in the 16–64 years age group)
Myopia	4%	
Retinal and choroidal degeneration	4%	(the second commonest cause in the 16–64 years age group)

Age

In developed nations malnutrition is not a significant problem; the treatment of infection is not dependent upon financial considerations, and therefore the prevalence of visual loss may be most effectively categorized according to the age of the individual. It must be emphasized that the following conditions are also major causes of blindness in the Third World, in addition to the burden of infection and malnutrition.

The Embryo
The developing individual is subjected to potential hazards from the moment of conception. The main problems in this category are hereditary eye disease and infection. Hereditary eye disease is considered in Chapter 16.

Infection during pregnancy, especially the first trimester, is of particular relevance to ocular maldevelopment. Rubella causes congenital cataracts and retinopathy, usually in association with cardiac defects and deafness, and congenital syphilis causes multiple systemic and ocular abnormalities, of which the most common are cataract and interstitial keratitis. These conditions are preventable by vaccination (rubella) or by antibiotic treatment to the mother prior to conception (syphilis) in most cases, but the emergence of the AIDS virus presents a new problem in the management of congenital eye disease.

The Neonate
Birth remains the greatest hurdle in life, although major advances in obstetrics and neonatology have reduced the risks in recent years. The retina has a limited capacity to survive ischaemia, and only for very short periods, so that any significant episode of anoxia during birth

causes irreparable damage. Conversely, excessive administration of oxygen post-partum, particularly in the premature infant, may precipitate retinopathy of prematurity (retrolental fibroplasia; see p. 122), with similarly disastrous consequences for the retina.

Childhood
The main causes of impaired vision in childhood are strabismic and deprivation amblyopia (due to squint and uncorrected refractive error, respectively) and trauma. However, these affect only one eye with rare exceptions. See Chapters 4 and 11.

The Working Population
This title is intended to incorporate all subjects between the ages of about 18 and 60 years. The commonest cause of visual loss in this group is diabetic eye disease. The ocular complications of diabetes are explained in Chapter 10, but it should be reiterated that the potentially disastrous ocular complications of diabetes are preventable or treatable (in the early stages) in most patients, given effective screening and management.

The other main cause of visual loss in this group is trauma, usually caused during manual occupations in which the wearing of protective glasses or goggles would have prevented the incident (e.g. hammering, lathe operating, or, less importantly, grinding), or by sport, of which squash ball injuries are undoubtedly the worst offender. Fortunately, trauma usually affects only one eye, but of course if the other eye has strabismic amblyopia, etc., the result is catastrophic for the individual.

The Elderly
The degenerative disorders of ageing affect the delicate tissues of the eye and thereby impair vision. The main causes of visual loss in this age group are macular degeneration, glaucoma and diabetic retinopathy (see pp. 112 and 208 and Chapters 5 and 10).

Cataract can be removed surgically, and, by the placing of an intraocular lens within the eye, excellent postoperative visual acuity and a wide field of vision are achieved in most patients. This operation has a high success rate, and cataract may therefore be regarded as a potentially curable condition.

Degenerative changes in the macular area of the retina produce early symptoms. Unfortunately, this is not amenable to cure, but it is essential to inform the patient that this condition affects only central vision, and will not usually progress to involve the peripheral fields. Most patients are understandably terrified of total blindness, and are usually relieved to be informed that their peripheral vision will not deteriorate. Although there is no cure for the condition, the patient's quality of life may be significantly improved by the provision of 'low-vision aids', instruments of high magnification that may be applicable for either near or distance vision or both. These are effective by utilizing the paramacular areas, but the major disadvantage of high magnification is constriction of the peripheral field of vision; for example, while reading, the patient may be able to see only a single word, or part of a word. Some patients are unable to cope with this restriction, but many are pleased to return to the joy of reading, even allowing for the difficulties of a restricted visual field.

The progression of glaucomatous ocular damage may be arrested — or at least retarded — by early diagnosis and treatment, described in Chapter 5.

INDEX

Note: Main page references are indicated in **bold**; page references to figures are in *italics*.